I0621547

THE
Lighthouse
PROJECT

A COLLECTIVE COMING HOME

The Lighthouse Project: A Collective Coming Home

Copyright © 2023 Soul Seed Legacy House

YGTMedia Co. Press Trade Paperback Edition

ISBN trade paperback: 978-1-998754-33-5

eBook: 978-1-998754-34-2

All Rights Reserved. No part of this book can be scanned, distributed, or copied without permission. This book or any portion thereof may not be reproduced or used in any manner whatsoever without the express written permission of the publisher at publishing@ygtmedia.co—except for the use of brief quotations in a book review.

The authors have made every effort to ensure the accuracy of the information within this book was correct at time of publication. The authors do not assume and hereby disclaim any liability to any party for any loss, damage, or disruption caused by errors or omissions, whether such errors or omissions result from accident, negligence, or any other cause. This book is not intended to be a substitute for the medical advice of a licensed physician. The reader should consult with their doctor in any matters relating to their health.

Published in Canada, for Global Distribution

by YGTMedia Co.

www.ygtmedia.co/publishing

To order additional copies of this book:

publishing@ygtmedia.co

Book design by Doris Chung

Cover design by Michelle Fairbanks

ePub & Kindle editions by Ellie Sipilä

Printed in North America

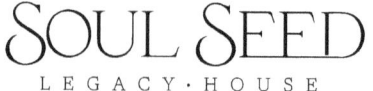

SOUL SEED

LEGACY·HOUSE

THE
Lighthouse
PROJECT

A COLLECTIVE COMING HOME

VOLUME 1

Sabrina Greer | Shantelle Bisson | Amanda Casinha
Preet Gill | Lindsay Lesage | Anita Rombough | Jessica Brasier
Apryl Jennings | Ashley Anne | Chernell Bartholomew
Lindsay Grace | Jessica Callery | Jenny Bitner | Nicole Campagna

Table of CONTENTS

Trigger Warning: suicide, sexual abuse/
assault, mental health, infertility

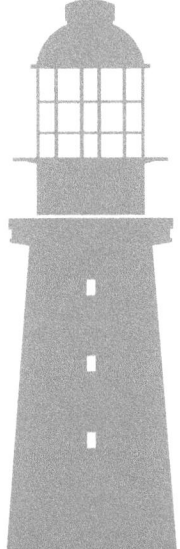

The Lighthouse

Sabrina Greer

The lighthouse stands tall and proud, head in the sky, a beacon
of light amid the storm.
She shines through the darkness and the rough and turbulent
waters; she is a symbol of hope as land takes form.
Some give up before her light breaks through, left floating
through the depths of the ocean evermore.
It is the most resilient who withstand the chaos to catch her
glimmer guiding them to shore.

—The Voice in My Soul

This poem channeled through me one evening. If you know anything about me, you know that I am not a poet. A writer, yes. An author, yes. A poet, no! The experience of channeled writing has been showing up for me more regularly since experiencing what I can only label as my "spiritual awakening," so I allow it to flow. I don't resist. I listen to the words and try to decode the messages. I *read* between the proverbial lines.

My interpretation of this verse, in particular, is that I have connections to the representations of the lighthouse. That I am on my own homecoming journey, rife with shadow work and deep healing ahead. I am also sure others have experienced the powerful symbolism of the lighthouse in their own stories. I bet this to myself, and the voice got louder.

Not unlike the repeating whispers in *Field of Dreams*, "If you build it, they will come," my little voice said, "Create the opportunity for them to share their hearts, and they will come." I threw the idea out to my editorial team and, of course, they were double thumbs-up in support. "What should I call it?" I asked my editorial manager with curiosity. Collectively, we decided to give it a working title, *The Lighthouse Project*, with the thought that a different title would drop in, in a channeled way, at a later time. I lobbed out the concept of *The Lighthouse Project: A Collective Coming Home* to our greater author community and on social media, and within five days, the book was full. Women I had never met felt "called" to the project. Dear friends and multi-published best-selling authors felt honored by the invitation. I was on to something. *The Lighthouse Project*—working title . . . or?

You know when you meet a child, let's call him Bob, and Bob clearly looks like a Joe. As you get to know Bob, however, you can't imagine another name. Bob it is. Same with *The Lighthouse Project*. The title stuck because it suits the mission. A collective coming home. Diverse recalls from brave humans sharing their raw and powerful stories of self-discovery: stories of resilience, self-acceptance, inner knowing, deep truth, and leaning into our own lighthouses, our intuition. It was a unanimous vote. Bob. *The Lighthouse Project*.

Chapter ONE

Frozen

Sabrina Greer

We need to be our own lighthouse and trust the beacon within will guide us safely to shore, even when we can't see the light.

@thesabrinagreer

Sabrina Greer

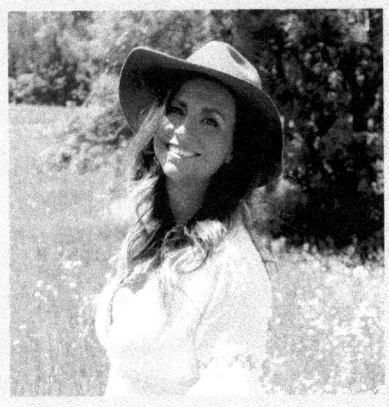

Sabrina Greer is a best-selling author, international publisher, motivational speaker, podcast host, and mentor to authors. She is the CEO and visionary behind YGTMedia Company and Soul Seed Legacy House, publishing imprints for thought leaders and creative entrepreneurs. A retired fashion model, Sabrina is passionate about positive body-image advocacy and self-love. She is a self-proclaimed "rookie farmer," as she raises a number of fur and feather babies alongside her three sons on a 70-acre farmstead in the woods. When Sabrina is not farming, momming, or running her businesses, you will likely find her at their lake house ferociously writing her memoir or reading a good nonfiction book!

INSTAGRAM @thesabrinagreer

To anyone riding the waves of ambiguous loss, I see you. This chapter is for you in hopes you find your lighthouse soon.

Frozen

We all experience storms we must weather. Every one of us, at some point, is tossed into rough and turbulent waters we must learn to navigate. How's your boat? Is it leaky and broken? Is it strong and capable? What materials did you use to build it? In case you missed the analogy, you're the boat. What tools are aboard to support you in the storm, because, as we know, there will always be darkness before the lighthouse turns on.

I've endured many rough waters in my forty years of life, both figuratively and literally, including in my yearlong stint as a yachty on the Mediterranean (we can save those stories for later, though). I very recently experienced my most violent and raging tempest to date. A storm so great that its wrath and total damage are still unknown. My boat was ill prepared for ice and snow, and it got stuck, unexpectedly, in the frozen ocean.

After much research and little discovery on the topic of my suffering, I came across a book by Pauline Boss called *Ambiguous Loss*. "Ambiguous loss makes us feel incompetent. It erodes our sense of mastery and destroys our belief in the world as a fair, orderly, and manageable place.

But if we learn to cope with uncertainty, we must realize that there are differing views of the world, even when that world is less challenged by ambiguity. . . . If we are to turn the corner and cope with uncertain losses, we must first temper our hunger for mastery. This is the paradox." She refers to this ambiguous loss as "frozen grief"—*finally, a cord to attach my sorrow to, two simple words to make sense of my suffering,* I thought.

What is frozen grief? To understand, we can break the term into the two parts. *Grief.* We've all experienced the deep pain and sorrow relating to the process of mourning something or someone lost, be it a loved one, a relationship, a former version of self, a pet. Grief is grief. That I know. I also know that regardless of what psychologists say about grief and its stages or steps, the grieving process is far from linear and is so unique to the person experiencing it.

Grief is like a tidal wave. It comes in strong and destructive, pulling you under to where you can no longer breathe. It's an undercurrent so intense that you lose control of your body. It's a force beyond measure. No matter how tightly you hold on, it drags you along the rough ocean floor, making you feel every tiny grain of sand as it tears your flesh, then pushes salt water into those fresh wounds.

Frozen grief is that same undercurrent and pain, but prolonged by uncertainty. Ambiguous loss is the kind that has no closure, no answers, no end. *Frozen.* In grief.

When I was five years old, my parents made the major life decision to become foster parents. Grieving the loss of her womb—the societal symbol of fertility and womanhood—and her ability to conceive again naturally, my mother, after five years with spirited little me, felt the inner knowing that she wanted to parent more children.

At first it wasn't easy. Babies would come and go, always staying long enough to take a sizable shard of our hearts with them. Small children would arrive, all hours of the day and night, soiled, abused, neglected, broken. I have clear memories of my exhausted mother in her rocking chair, bottle-feeding colicky infants as they screamed and spit up in her face. I remember the hours she spent with her ear attached to our rotary phone, talking to social workers, therapists, and specialists, advocating as best she could for her new offspring. Then there were the supervised visits with disgruntled biological families and the endless appointments and drop-ins. I always admired my mom for her ability to somehow stay calm amid the utter chaos.

My mother eventually found her footing, grounding herself in the pride and fulfillment that fostering provided her. It is truly a thankless job (as parenting often is). It was a 24/7/365 commitment to the protection and well-being of others, with the added layer of having so many unknowns, ranging needs, and limited resources.

On a cold day in January 1988, we got the call: an emergency placement would be delivered that day, a little boy. His backstory looked a little something like this: teenage mother, possible substance user, negligence and abuse suspected, infant found alone, crying, broken arm and potential internal bleeding, immediate care to follow medical analysis. My parents knew the drill. While my father was the silent supporter, he was always there in the peripheral, making sure there was food on the table and a roof over our heads. My mom thrived in the madness; it felt like a movie where the detective (my mom) had to solve the case studies before the children arrived. She would pre-diagnose medical conditions and speculate the situations of the biological parents as we ran around the house making sure the nursery met Children's Aid

Society standards. Bottles sanitized, check. Fresh bedding and towels, check. Everything childproofed, check.

That evening, Geoffrey Allen arrived at our home. He had big blue eyes, a head full of blond hair, and the largest hands I've ever seen on a baby. Even though his circumstances were far from ideal, he was happy and full of smiles. His little baby cast and sling supported his broken arm and punctured lung. It was the first time I experienced chosen love; love beyond the bloodline of my parents. From that moment on, Geoffrey became Justin, because he was "just in time" as my mother said. At that time I didn't know what he was in time for, but I now believe he was just in time to breathe the life into my family that my mother had been longing for.

Eighteen months later we adopted Justin, and six-year-old me even got to sign the legal papers. Like with a marriage license, I vowed to love this human as long as we both should live. I swore to protect and guide him for as long as my heart produced a beat. I proudly and excitedly, with conviction and deep love, chose my brother that day. I was officially a sister.

We had a humble and beautiful upbringing. We lived in a suburban bungalow with a big backyard close to a park on the water where we would feed the birds or play on the playground. Our safe little street always smelled of lilacs even though we were less than a kilometer from the nuclear power plant. Every day felt like a birthday party, between all the neighbors' kids, cousin playdates, and dozens of foster kids that came and went. But the constant was always Justin and me. We were inseparable.

When he was a baby, he was *my* baby. I slept in his crib, gave him his bottles, cleaned up his messes, pushed him in the stroller, changed him, bathed him, and loved him wholeheartedly. He never left my sight. As he learned to toddle and walk, I was there to hold his hand and catch his falls. His first word was "Bwina," which he would continue to call me for most of our childhood, even once his consonants formed.

When he was three years old, we discovered his anaphylaxis to bee stings through a near-death encounter of blue lips, closed airway, and body convulsions. From that day onward, I walked in front of him by about six feet and flailed my body aggressively onto bees' nests and hives so they would sting me and not my baby brother. I've always had a flair for the dramatic, and I had vowed to protect him, always. His health struggles heightened with every birthday, and we soon unearthed an array of allergies, asthma, and other ailments. I spent many days and nights by his side, in his hospital crib, and later, bed. I always lovingly thought of my brother as a glass jar. It would take every ounce of energy and effort to fill him up, but the glass would often shatter, leaving us all depleted.

I left home when I was sixteen to see the world and chase my dreams as an international fashion model. Justin was barely eleven, and it was the first time since he was six months old that we were apart for more than a few days. I was hesitant to leave my baby bro, so I took all necessary measures to remain close: I sent handwritten letters and postcards from every country, and I made sure I came home for family holiday gatherings. He was always so proud of me and in awe of my travels and accomplishments, and he loved hearing stories of foreign lands. And middle school was promising for him—he loved sharing his sports trophies and academic awards with me even more.

As Justin entered high school, my modeling contracts got longer and farther away from home. Japan for six months, Italy for eight, South Africa for ten months, back to Spain for three. We inevitably grew apart. I loved hearing about his straight As in school and collection of sports awards and accolades. He defied the odds when it came to athletics. Volleyball, basketball, baseball, high jump, long jump, relay . . . you name it, he was at the top of the game. The once-frail, asthmatic, little glass jar developed into a six foot six unbreakable machine who his teammates referred to as "Stretch" on the courts and in the fields. He was unstoppable. He had caught an epic wave and rode it through with vigor and pride. Until he crashed. No wave lasts forever.

✳ ✳ ✳

"I think that's your phone, babe," my husband grumbled, placing his phone back on the nightstand.

"Huh? What time is it?" I groggily responded.

"Midnight, I think," he said as he rolled over with a faint snore.

I closed my eyes with the knowledge that my children were asleep in their beds and they were my only responsibility. It was likely one of my clients on the other side of the world, a.k.a. Australia, and it could wait until the morning. Morning wake-ups at 6:30 arrive far too quickly from midnight, but that is what time our days begin. Breakfast, backpacks, lunches, school drop-offs, hubby out the door to work. Every morning feels like a sweet little hurricane before Mama (that's me) gets to breathe her first breath of calm and take that delicious first sip of hot coffee. In the chaos of our typical morning routine, some days I don't look at my phone until after drop-off; this was one of those days.

I opened my messages, excited to see what my clients in Australia had to say the night before.

"Hey, are you Justin's sister?" a strange man I'd never seen or met before asked. I read further. "I'm worried about him. He sent me these messages last night, and he seems serious." I scrolled down to the screen-shots of a conversation between this man and my brother. To summarize their texts, it had gotten dark enough that my brother wanted to leave this place, and the plan was to do so by suicide that night. I thanked the kind stranger as I jumped into my car.

"Nine-one-one, what's your emergency?" A voice on the line echoed through my hands-free.

"My br . . . brother . . . might be dead." I don't remember much more of the conversation, but the police and paramedics arrived several minutes before me. We met in the front yard of the house where he lived in the basement apartment.

Justin and I hadn't spoken for nearly a year. His behavior had become incredibly destructive in ways that I could not support, and I had to make the very challenging decision as a mother to three young boys to separate him from our world. Telling my brother, the uncle to my children and half of my heart, that he was no longer welcome in my life had been the tip of the iceberg. Now this?

"Does he have any weapons? Is he armed or dangerous?" a very aggressive, bearded man in uniform yelled at me.

"What? I don't know. If he's even alive, I very much doubt he is moving."

What felt like hours later, but was mere moments, they took my brother by ambulance to the hospital—breathing, heart beating, alive. Unrecognizable to me.

Here I was, forty years old, by his hospital bedside again, this time not for bee stings and asthma attacks, though. His eyes, still big and blue. Behind the tears, I heard him say "Bwina," and I wept. I wept as he slept off the poison he had consumed. "Enough to kill a horse," they said. I wept because even though he was technically alive, I knew the journey ahead would be treacherous.

As an adult, Justin has had to weather many storms of his own. Substance abuse. Addiction. Homelessness. Countless informal (and formal) mental health diagnoses, and many more challenges that aren't my place to share. I don't know why this happens to some people. I guess some get lost before the lighthouse turns on. I don't know why our health system is so incredibly reactive instead of proactive.

I often wonder if his foul weather began when I removed the umbrella I had been holding above his head for most of his life. He got stung once I stopped jumping into beehives. He forgot how to swim when I left with the life preserver. We can't do this, though: blame ourselves, however tempting. We all need to build our own boat. Watching someone you love so deeply destroy themselves is an emotional tsunami. Not knowing from day to day or moment to moment where they are, whether they are alive and hurting, if it's bad news buzzing on your phone—that is the ice storm. Frozen. In grief.

Boats aren't made for frozen waters. It was an iceberg that sank the *Titanic*, after all. We need to go beyond building a strong boat—we need wings and scuba gear and an all-season, indestructible flying submarine that can support us through any storm. We need to be our own lighthouse and trust the beacon within will guide us safely to shore, even when we can't see the light. My brother is still in his raging storm, without a boat. He is gasping for air and barely treading water, and I pray every day that he'll see the light and fight like hell to build his boat and get to safety.

Chapter TWO

Friendship: The Ups, the Downs, and the Beauty Left Behind

Shantelle Bisson

Instinctively, I knew in order to build a circle, I needed a starting point, and that starting point was me.

@shantellebisson @withoutlosingyourcool

Shantelle Bisson

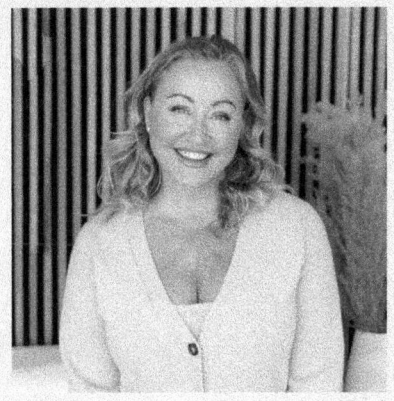

Shantelle Bisson is a two-time best-selling author, keynote speaker, and founder of the Without Losing Your Cool movement. She was born and raised in Toronto and splits her time between Toronto and the Kawartha region of northern Ontario at her marina, Shantilly's Place, that she purchased in 2018. Along with being an author and producer, Shantelle, a recovering actress, has three beautiful daughters and two four-legged kids with husband, Yannick Bisson, star of Canada's number one drama series, CBC's Murdoch Mysteries. Shantelle is currently in production on the fourth season of her weekly podcast, *Without Losing Your Cool*.

INSTAGRAM @shantellebisson @withoutlosingyourcool

To all the friendships I've had along the way: the ones who stayed, and the ones who came and went but left their beauty on my heart. Your lessons were invaluable, and I'm grateful for our time together.

Friendship: The Ups, the Downs, and the Beauty Left Behind

We come into this world whole. Secure in ourselves. Not knowing or needing the approval of anybody else. Yes, we need to be nurtured by parents; we need to be fed, held, and loved. But we don't *need* anything else. Not approval. Not acceptance. Not a massive circle of people in our lives to make our lives, or us, *whole.*

Then that all changes. We leave the nest and begin to socialize; we learn about external relationships that bring us joy, that enrich our lives and our spirits. These new and wonderful relationships are called *friendships.*

We run home from school and share with our parents, our siblings, anybody within earshot, how much we love our new friends. Our lives become fuller and richer as we learn from them, grow from them, and discover new things about ourselves, and the world at large. Friendships are incredible. We feel and we develop, subconsciously, a deep sense of gratitude for our expanded worlds. Our friends become intertwined into the fabrics of our day-to-day lives. Many of us might start to change the way we dress, or develop new ideas, or, as in my case, even start to change the way we behave. This might be good or not so good depending on the friends one surrounds themselves with. Our friends, we start to learn, have a massive impact on us, and as we grow up and head into our teen years, we perhaps remember our parents/caregivers warning us about certain other kids, and we may not understand the *why* because we're not fully developed emotionally.

When I was little, my parents were on and off. They had an incredibly volatile, tumultuous marriage, likely due to my father's alcoholism and his habitual infidelity. Life was anything but stable for me. But here's the cool thing about being little . . . I didn't *know* that the screaming matches and the violence that my dad inflicted—verbally and sometimes physically—weren't normal. I had nothing else to compare my life to. How could I? I was just a little girl. It wasn't until my circle expanded through friendship that I came to learn that other girls my age were not dealing with the same bullshit at home that I was, and that's when things began to change for me. The longing for "normal" became a thing I dreamed about, a thing I longed for, and a thing I never, ever thought I would have.

Friendship opens our eyes, which is why we have to be careful who we allow inside our inner, most sacred circle. Because of the reality of my family situation, my mom always had to make sure that she could afford to house and feed us for the inevitable moment in time when my father would need to leave the family home. My mom found a cute three-bedroom apartment for us. My brothers shared a room, I had my own, and she and Dad had theirs. The first memory I have of this apartment building was how many other kids our age there were. It was like summer camp! There were just so many kids. Boys, girls, other sisters and brothers, and we all hung out together. It was easy. There was no drama. There was only laughter, joy, and ease. These friends all made my life richer and fuller, and they certainly distracted me from what was happening at home, which I was beginning to learn was anything but normal.

I was nine and I loved this thing called friendship.

Until I didn't.

I vividly recall that summer when everything changed. I started to develop breasts, and the boys who had been friends, who would pick me to be on their team for Red Rover or race me in climbing trees, started to leer at me. Started to pull me into dark corners when we'd all be hanging out together, to grope me and try to kiss me. This rolled over into school as well. The girls who used to play hopscotch and jump rope with me started to dwindle. They wouldn't eat lunch with me anymore. Suddenly I was all alone. Suddenly girls would follow me home to push me, to call me names, and to make my life a new kind of hell. Suddenly there was no longer a huge friend group, there were only one or two friends left standing, and my once large, stable social circle became very, very, very small. And I remember feeling pain on a whole new level during those two years between ages nine and eleven when in my childhood mind I began to believe that I must be the problem.

I must be unlikeable.

I felt all alone, as if no one wanted to be friends with me anymore. Which felt pretty awful. Even now, when I close my eyes, I remember how sad and lost I felt. And as a young girl, the only survival mechanism I had was to disown myself in order to "fit in" in the hopes that I would once again have friends, which began my journey of living outside myself so I would never be alone again. I betrayed myself to hopefully find like-minded people to be friends with.

I tried soccer in the hopes of finding soccer friends. I didn't.

I joined a softball team, believing I would find friends there, but didn't. I came up empty. Every new box I tried to fit myself into, hoping to find friends there, came up empty. None of this stopped the bullying. I was still being left out, and my heart still hurt like hell. Looking back now, as an adult, I understand that I wasn't finding any new friends because I was being a chameleon. By trying to change who I was with the hope and desire that if I became what others wanted me to be, they would like me. I was being inauthentic. How could I have possibly known as a young girl that the reason why I was having trouble making friends was likely due to the fact that I was being fake. Even kids can spot a phony from a mile away. I was trying to find like-minded people, but to who? Not me. Because none of these activities I was engaging in while trying to find new friends were things that I cared one damn thing about. I eventually stopped trying to change myself to fit in and was happy that I had a couple very good girlfriends to get me through. There were times, while witnessing others have huge friend groups and always having something to do on the weekends, when I felt a pang of loneliness and did wish I was liked and that I fit in.

Life carried on, as it is known to do, and I entered junior high alone and scared. Scared because within weeks of arriving there—there being a new school in a relatively new neighborhood—we had moved so I could start again because a group of boys from my previous elementary school tried to rape me in my home. (But that, my friends, is a different story that I share in my book *Loving Yourself Without Losing Your Cool*, so no need to retell it here.) A very strange thing happened to me in this new, nice, "safe" part of the city: the school bully decided she was going to kick my ass.

Why? Well, nobody knew. Apparently, this was just what this girl did. She picked girls she didn't like (mind you, she also didn't know them) and would beat them up. And word in the hallways was that I was going to be that girl for her.

That's when I decided. Absolutely not. I was not going to be her literal punching bag. So, I set out to win her over. To become her best friend so that I could "stay alive" in this new environment that didn't feel anything like the warmth and joy of what friendship had started out being for me. The way I became the best friend and not the victim of this girl is that I beat her at her own game. I, too, became a bully. I surveyed my new school, the new group of girls, and like a lioness, I figured out one of the weaker ones and started to pick on her. (Looking back now, my stomach turns, and I send out my most sincere apologies to the young girl who was my victim. If you happen to remember me, please know that I am truly and deeply sorry for how I abused you as I looked to save myself at all costs.)

Survival of the fittest.

This was beginning to be a recurring theme in my young life. That and "trust no one." Not your friends, as they'll assault you. Not the girls, as they'll turn on you. Not your family, as they won't protect you (my rape and sexual abuse took place in the "safety" of my family). No one was to be trusted. And if I wanted to be safe, I had to not be myself. So, I became different. I became what I needed to be in order to be safe.

And my plan to become safe in my new environment as quickly as possible worked. It wasn't very long until the Queen Bee was my best friend. Before I knew it, we were bullying other girls together. We were smoking, lying, and sneaking around, and when I tell you it didn't feel very good at all to become somebody I wasn't, that would be an understatement. Because it felt downright awful.

Years came and went. I continued to move through my life adjusting who I was in order to not be bullied, to not be picked on, to not be left all alone on the outside of life looking in. I wish I could type the words to you that I eventually fell back into a beautiful friend group, or that I enjoyed the experience of a large group of girlfriends who grew up together, who went to university together, who got married and stood up for one another, and who are now godmothers to each other's children, but that's not what happened for me. Now, I don't want to leave you with the impression that I was in my late thirties sitting all alone in my home with no one to love or be loved by. That is far from the reality of my life. I had a husband who I loved madly, three wonderful daughters who kept me busy, and my life was full. I had a beautiful relationship with my mom, and I had three very good friends: one being my best friend from my first year of high school, one being a girlfriend I gained and fell in love with in my early twenties (we were both living in New Zealand while our husbands filmed a television show together), and one who has been my friend since the day she started dating my youngest brother. (She married him almost thirty years ago.)

Friendship is a beautiful thing, and I definitely felt fortunate to have the three deep and trusted relationships that I had. There are some people who could make friends with a rattlesnake, while others, like me, are a bit more cautious about who they let into their inner circle. For me, I tended to keep my circle smaller, and I always have (rightfully so, given my past). But in the back of my mind there was that desire to have more friends, like I'd had before. Because when there are small kids involved, and a busy husband, two friends in one city, and one in another country, they don't always meet your needs. Besides, meeting all your emotional needs is a lot to place on the shoulders of three women. From what I witnessed in high school, and as a young mom, I not only knew that I could have more, but I also craved more. I don't subscribe to the notion that we "must settle" in life. The "take what you get and be happy with it" mindset is not one I think we need to live by. I mean, ONE LIFE people, what are you waiting for?

I remember reading an article on Cameron Diaz where she talked on and on and on ad nauseam about her "sisterhood": how she had this massive circle of loving, kind, supportive women in her life who enriched it, that were in her corner no matter what, and how magical and essential that was to her well-being, and I felt ripped off. I distinctly remember a short moment after reading the article when I closed my eyes and wondered what on earth that would actually feel like.

I wanted to feel that.

I wanted to have that.

When I closed my eyes and traveled back in time to my childhood, the core memories that flooded back were all the things that Cameron described having as an adult. And I was determined to get back to all that juicy goodness. I was committed to never being an island again. Maybe you can relate to what I'm sharing, and you may be wondering to yourself, *how do so many women still have those childhood friends, while I have just one?* I'm not talking about liking my best friend from Grade 4's Instagram posts, I'm talking about friends who still live near each other, who are raising their families together, and who go on family trips together. There are tons of women out there who have this life, but maybe, like me, you're not one of them. So where are they? How do you find a new circle? How do you create an inclusive group of women to lean on, to rely on, to *trust* with all the pieces of you that make you, *you*, if you don't even know who you are?

Well, an excellent place to start is by looking in the mirror. Which is precisely what I did. So began my journey of creating it for myself. Instinctively, I knew in order to build a circle, I needed a starting point, and that starting point was me. First, I needed to put myself back together. First, I needed to strip away all the falsities I had created while I was busy for two decades trying to be what I thought others wanted me to be in order to like me. How could anybody ever like me if I didn't like myself? If I had fabricated a personality that wasn't mine? Who were they even becoming friends with, if not me?

I was living inside myself but outside of my true self.

I started to do deep intense healing work on myself, uncovering all the layers of protection I had placed upon my shiny sparkly self to dim my light—to play small, to "fit in" so that I wouldn't stand out. Because what I had learned out in the world was shining bright brought jealousy, envy, and ugliness with it. Playing small allowed me to sneak past the haters. But what I also learned about playing small was that it destroyed my heart. It left me longing. It left me living my one life as a spectator of it rather than an active participant in it. And that would NOT do. I would not steal my one chance for a big, brilliant, bold, and magical life to please people who didn't matter to me as much as I mattered to me. So, I stopped. I gave it up. I let it all go, and I let myself back in. I welcomed Shantelle back into herself, and a beautiful thing happened shortly after that. I found my people. I found my sisterhood.

Now, it wasn't a straight line to my people, and it likely won't be for you either. There were a lot of trials and tribulations along my way to finding my sisterhood. Some failed starts, if you will. Friendship, like any other intimate relationship in your life, requires you to devote the time needed to foster it; quite frankly, there are times in our lives when, whether due to our demanding careers or having a young family, it's not possible to add anybody new to our circle of friends. I'm not talking about acquaintances here. I'm talking about "ride-or-dies." I'm talking about the type of friendship where you can tell them absolutely anything about yourself and know that they will take it to their graves. These sorts of friendships don't happen in a single day, which means that if you're in the middle of an insanely busy personal time of your life, it will be more challenging to expand your group. Sometimes it can be due to a job change that takes you out of your home city or having little kids who have you living life like some sort of professional juggler. There are so many reasons why our friendships, as women, ebb and flow. And not all of them need be rooted in past friendship trauma.

It took me well into my forties to really be available on a soul level to myself and to others, and then a beautiful thing happened: I found a whole bunch of fascinating, inspiring women from all sorts of backgrounds, both culturally and socioeconomically, who I became friends with, and each one of them has taught me a great number of things. Some stayed for a short time, others remained for a long time, and then others, four to be exact, remain today. Four more added to that deep inner circle where truths of fears, dreams, victories, and losses are shared. Where trust is sacred and honored.

I have found my long desired "sisterhood" that Cameron spoke of. I have built myself a group of seven wonderful women.

Women to cry with.
Women to laugh with.
Women to be silent with.
Women to travel with.

Women to build with.
Women to hold up, and sometimes to be held up by.

At long last, at the age of fifty-four, I have my people. I have returned home to the purity of that young girl who enjoyed friendship with ease. With joy. With trust and by faith. But it's not to say that these relationships are without conflict, or sometimes pain and upset, as that would be some bizarre, fake, shallow existence. No. These friendships are filled with complexities, and it sometimes takes days/weeks/months of drifting apart while we figure out within ourselves how to resolve an issue that has shown up in the relationship. It's not a reason to quit the friendship but rather an opportunity to dig deeper and uncover another layer of intimacy between each other as we simultaneously uncover a deeper connection to self.

Remember this: it is never too late to expand your circle of support, inspiration, love, and strength by way of friendship. Be open to the joy of building new relationships, without any expectations. You might invest years into a friend who feels like they will be with you until the end, only to learn that you've grown apart—not due to any disagreement or drama, but simply because they came and gave you exactly what you needed at that time in your life, and you did the same for them in return.

When it comes to girlfriends, it isn't how long they've known you, it's about how deeply you connect and what you give to one another during your stay together. Friendship is about quality, not quantity, so as long as you're giving and receiving what you need in your friend relationships, then, just like any other intimate relationship in your life, there is no need to go looking for more just for the sake of it. When you stand firmly in the knowing of self, you can have a deeper confidence in your value as a human in your relationships with others, but most importantly, in your relationship with yourself. And trust me when I say that your friendship to yourself is the most important one you will ever have, so please make sure that you nurture that one the most.

Chapter THREE

Permission to Grieve

Amanda Casinha

Once you give yourself permission to grieve, the grief journey is yours and yours alone, and no one can define that for you.

@ThatTorontoMom @GrindSocialMedia

Amanda Casinha

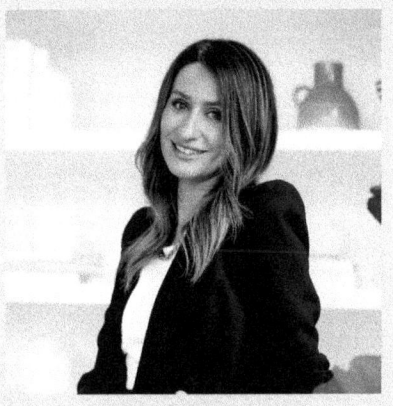

Amanda Casinha founded Grind Social Media + Co., a full-service social media marketing and consulting agency. After building a seven-figure business in her twenties, she is now passionate about using her fifteen-plus years in marketing to help other businesses grow online. She is a best-selling published author, speaker, Toronto Mom Influencer, and podcast host. Amanda has always been a community-minded advocate. She has spent her free time being involved with the Toronto Distress Centres, fundraising for women's shelters and the homeless in Toronto, and mentoring numerous women entrepreneurs through Mamas and Co. You can find her drinking coffee and listening to true crime podcasts when she isn't watching bad reality TV. She spends her time living between Toronto and Portugal with her husband and two beautiful daughters.

INSTAGRAM @ThatTorontoMom @GrindSocialMedia

To Phil, Felipa, and Lola, for showing me what love is again.

Permission to Grieve

The sun is glistening across the Atlantic, and my children are running across the sand with their newfound friends. I look over at my husband and think about how lucky I am to be spending my summers in Europe with our family—the dream we envisioned almost seventeen years ago is finally here.

It was no small feat to make this come together (work and travel with two toddlers is no joke), but just as my parents did with my sister and me, we were steadfast in making it happen. Being here is where I feel the most like myself: "carefree, go with the flow, don't need to control everything" Amanda.

I'm the mother I have always wanted to be: one that isn't fueled with rage at the smallest inconvenience, one that has patience for her partner, and one that can lean on others for support. It was a long road home, one that I didn't think I would see in my lifetime after all that had happened. Maybe it's the air, maybe it's the European laid-back lifestyle, maybe it's all just coming together since I've had time to just sit and breathe and grieve. I am finally home. I have finally given myself permission—permission to be fully who I am, permission to accept that I can have a good life, permission to grieve.

The Path of Grief Resistance

"She died too soon." A phrase I had heard countless times.

"I can't believe this happened."

"I know, right? Why would she do this?"

If I knew, then maybe it wouldn't be the only thing consuming my brain every second of the day. "What happened?"

Hard stop.

When I was nineteen years old, my mother died by suicide. It was the worst day of my life. The life that I knew was just gone. I would never be the same person. This realization was a bittersweet moment that I can look back on now after almost two decades and understand that this was supposed to be my path in life. Without this loss, I would have never worked with other survivors of suicide, I would have never become involved in a community raising awareness for an important cause, I probably wouldn't have my own family to prove that I could do it differently, and I wouldn't be the me that I am so proud of now—a resilient and empathetic woman.

The details of how she died aren't important, they never were. When you lose someone, you can try and understand the *why* all you want, but here's the thing you never will: whether by suicide or physical illness, there are so many circumstances around the loss, and you can try and make sense of why this all happened, but your fundamental beliefs will be challenged, and you are left to grieve it all.

I tried to ignore my grief; I did it really well for the majority of my twenties, or I thought I did. That period of my life was a blur, and to be honest, I don't remember most of it. From binge drinking and partying to just flat out being in denial about all of it, I wanted to forget, so I pushed it all down. What I didn't realize was that all that grief was presenting itself in physical and emotional ways.

Grief can present itself in very complex ways, and I was basically the poster child of complicated grief. I felt rage, anger, guilt, shame, rejection, sadness, and fear. In looking back now, I was really fucking afraid. Would I end up the same way? The emotional distress that I was ignoring then manifested into a diagnosis of insomnia—I just didn't sleep, ever. Until I started to deal with it all.

Death by suicide makes many people uncomfortable, something I learned very quickly. When I look back on other deaths I experienced, everyone was around—everyone made the time and effort to ask how I was doing and stuck by my side. When someone dies by suicide, however, you learn who is going to stay by your side and who isn't. I learned later in life that this was their grieving process and that no one is going to grieve the same way as I was. There is no right way to grieve. And I had to accept that quickly. I wasn't abandoned, they were just dealing with their own grief.

My life changed when I finally decided to stop the self-destruction and gave myself permission to feel. There was a clarity about why I was put on this earth, something I had been questioning from the day my mom died. Finding a therapist that specialized in complicated grief was the best gift I could give myself. I learned that my anger and extreme feelings of guilt were normal. I learned that I could be happy and extremely depressed at the same time. That while grieving this loss, they could exist together.

I was learning that relationships were going to change because I had changed. I looked at the world differently, and so I looked at the people in my world differently. The small things that used to unite us no longer did. The bigger problems they had didn't seem to matter to me anymore, so I let go of some important relationships in my life because they just no longer aligned with who I was becoming. I learned that I didn't need to feel guilty for letting go of them, that it was healthy and normal to move on.

When you learn that grief doesn't ever go away, it can feel like you will always be angry and sad, but then you learn that you will build a toolbox for all the emotions. You can open it up and pull from it whenever you need it. You learn quickly what works and what doesn't; who you can lean on and who you can't. Once that sunk in, it was freeing. I was never going to get over her death, but I could choose to get through it, one day at a time.

The Road to Motherhood

I still catch myself thinking about what life would look like if my mom hadn't died. If she was still here. She was my constant, the one who provided stability and direction. She guided the storms and led the way forward. Then she was gone. My world was ripped from under me as a young nineteen-year-old: all the love, comfort, and security I knew was gone with one action that I could not control. My mother took her own life. And when she did, I lost a part of myself that I would not find again until I became a mother myself.

The road to motherhood was not an easy one. It took many years and failed attempts at pregnancy. We were frustrated and disappointed, and I was lonely. I had my friends to speak to, but I didn't have my mom. There was something really rage inducing and isolating about going through infertility without the person who gave life to you. I couldn't ask any questions about health history, I had nothing to compare it against, and I had to trust in the doctors to figure it out.

After three years of trying, we finally decided to go the IVF route and had our date to start: June 1. As we approached the day, I was nervous and carefree; we might finally have the child we had been wishing for. And then on May 23, the anniversary of my mother's death, I was out with my best friend when we started chatting about menstrual cycles, and I realized that it had been a while since I'd had one—I was really carefree at this point. I stopped at the drugstore and picked up six pregnancy tests (one cannot be too sure). I remember laughing to myself and thinking, *Mom, if this is your idea of a joke, thank you.*

I ended up walking the ten blocks home, and in that time, all the emotions hit me. Was it grief? Relief? Who knew, I was just anxious to get home to take those tests. And I did, all six of them. Two lines appeared quickly. My husband was on a work trip and unavailable for three hours, so I sat on my couch and laughed in disbelief. Then I picked up my phone with the immediate urge to look for my mom's phone number, a number that hadn't existed for more than a decade. For a fleeting second I almost let the grief through, the anger that was boiling inside of me, but I didn't—it would have to wait. It was a reality that I didn't want to face, so I buried it and waited to call my husband.

When our daughter arrived, it was one of the best days of my life, and it was also one of the worst. I immediately wanted to share her with the only person I physically couldn't, so I did the second-best thing: I named my firstborn after her, and then I buried the grief more deeply.

We had limited help with our daughter due to a variety of circumstances, and with this came resentment toward my husband. He got to leave and go to work and gasp!—talk to adults, take real breaks, and not be a human food machine. We had to work really hard on our relationship during this time. It took therapy and angry conversations on both of our parts to feel heard. We were surprised when our second daughter was conceived, as it was during a time when our relationship was rocky. Another incredible moment that my grief stole from me.

The grief had taken over. I was angry, stressed out, and envious of any friend with a mother who helped them. I couldn't stand to hear the stories of how they had help, even though my family was still helping when they could. I smiled through, my teeth clenched when they complained that their mothers were always in their space. I would have given anything to have her in the way. When they complained that their moms were trying to give advice and parent for them, I quietly thought about how incredible it would be to have someone to ask questions to and to be intrusive. I thought about how incredible it would be to just pick up the phone to call her when I was having a hard time, or to just fall into her arms when I was exhausted. I just couldn't believe that this was my life, that this was happening to me. I was fucking furious. Not at my friends, as they were incredible. I was just so furious that this was my life and what I thought would be the best part of my life, motherhood, was ruined. But what I refused to acknowledge was that it was all the grief from years of suppression and fighting to get out.

You see, I learned that grief and all the important things we put off are just like big stones. And our brain and being are like red wagons. Don't ask me why they're red, they just are. And every time we put an emotion or thing aside that we don't want to deal with, the wagons get another stone added. And they get harder to pull. You get a little slower. And then another emotion or avoidance equals another stone.

And then another, and another. Eventually, you run out of space. Your wagons are too heavy. They stop. They can't go any further. Then they knock you down, leaving you on the ground helpless with a giant mess to clean up.

No one tells you how hard motherhood is going to be. No one tells you that one day your mom will die and you won't have her there to support you through a new part of your life when you need her the most. You're told how magical and wonderful the experience is, that you will truly fall into place and know who you are at that moment. But that wasn't my experience. My emotions were intense, the way I approached motherhood was questioned and judged, and I was dealing with all this through an extreme moment of grieving in my life, all while consuming myself with my daughters, taking in every first moment, being amazed by the fact that I'd brought two perfect beings into existence. When I had a good day, I relished it because it gave me the strength for the bad ones.

The idea that the one person you want to be there with you through these big firsts, these big momentous occasions, couldn't be there was all too much some days. How could I be so happy when my mother was gone and would never get to experience the joy of her granddaughters? The survivor's guilt was real. I was so happy and yet crumbling inside at every single moment that she was missing.

I had to learn to deal with these emotions as they came up and to have important conversations with and to lean on my family and friends for support. And it was hard. But I owed it to my children, and I owed it to myself. I really wanted to keep filling those stupid red wagons because that was easier. For me, there was no option, and in the moment when I started to set boundaries, to ask for help, and to literally scream into a pillow when I was angry, I started to feel lighter—the wagons weren't working against me anymore.

The Journey Home

The road to get to where I am today was long and winding, with obstacles at every turn: having to choose me in a world where selfishness is frowned upon; learning that the care I needed to give to myself was self-care and not selfish; knowing that working on myself made me a better friend, partner, and mother; becoming unapologetically myself when I was so used to pleasing everyone else in fear that they, too, would leave me.

Losing a mother doesn't happen in a moment; it takes years to fully realize what the impact is. There is an emptiness inside of me, a void yet to be filled, because no one will truly love me like my mother did. I am still grieving. I am still working through some very complicated emotions. I am soon approaching the age that my mother was when she died, something that brings up some serious unresolved issues. Until this point, I've been mirroring and reflecting on who she was, what was happening physically for her. When this day comes, I will have officially lived longer without her than with her.

In the past, I would have gone through this alone. I would've used my anger against those who love me, I would've pushed them away to protect myself, I would've thought that I had no support. I know now that this isn't reality. I can create whatever it is that I want and need to help me get through this. And that is exactly what I will do.

For a long time I wouldn't celebrate anything: birthdays, graduations, anything really. Now I find myself celebrating more and bringing in old traditions that my mom would have been so happy to be a part of. While it's still hard, I am choosing to move forward and give my children the experiences I had.

Grief is complicated. There is no right or wrong way to grieve. I can't guarantee anything in life, but I will say this: the pain you are feeling right this second is temporary, and it will probably get worse before it gets better. Relish the good days, as they will give you the strength for the bad ones. You will get through this and don't let anyone ever tell you to get over it. Take your time, on your own time. Once you give yourself permission to grieve, the grief journey is yours and yours alone, and no one can define that for you.

So, I sit here on the beach in Europe, the same spot she sat in every summer while watching us play. Now I am doing the same; I'm watching my kids run in the sand and splash in the ocean. And while she isn't here to witness it, I can feel her presence, and I am relishing it. It's a good day. It will get me through the hard ones to come.

Chapter FOUR

The Many Truths of Anger

Preet Gill

As I process and integrate
the many truths of anger,
I can feel its alchemizing
power working within me.
Forgiveness, compassion,
and peace rise to the
surface.

@preet.k.gill

Preet Gill

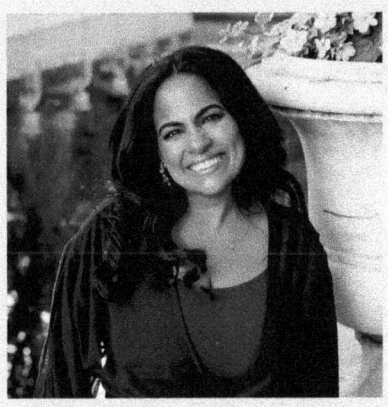

Preet Gill has always been drawn to guiding and healing, beginning her career as a Social Worker, and later in life as a Kundalini Yoga Instructor, Reiki Practitioner, Somatic Breathwork Facilitator, and Akashic Records Guide. She blends these empowering healing modalities, along with her own life experience of alchemizing big T and little t traumas, as an Intuitive Soul Guide and Transformation Coach for her clients to step into vibrant, radiant energy, tap into their inner wisdom, and uncover their deeper life purpose. Preet adores reading, stargazing, and travel adventures—experiences that cultivate the delicious, expansive feelings of curiosity, wonder, and awe. She is a mama to two lovely and lively daughters, is in a loving marriage, and is surrounded by a circle of beautiful beings. Cacao, all things coconut, and '90s' hip-hop and reggae speak to her soul.

INSTAGRAM @preet.k.gill

To my father, Charanjit Singh Gill. Thank you, dear Dad, for guiding me on this soul path of truth, reclamation, and zest for life. I miss you and I love you. Now, let's put on the old Panjabi tunes and jam.

The Many Truths of Anger

I wake with a start. My breath ragged and eyes large, unfocused. I feel heat around me, yet shiver. I close my eyes, slowing my breath. Watching the dancing flames behind my eyelids, I relax and sink back into the darkness of the night and softness of my pillow. Another dream visit with Goddess Pele (pronounced Peh-Leh), a deity of fire, lightning, and volcanoes.

It started with dreams of a mountainous island with active volcanoes and lush rainforest. It is a land I had not visited in this lifetime, but it felt familiar, vivid, and known. A land that has been calling for some time. One that feels like I have walked upon her soil and shared in her secrets. A few years ago, I looked up active volcanic islands, and Hawaii's Big Island came up. It has the most volcanic activity in the world. From the images on the internet, it looked so similar to the place of my dreams. But Hawaii is part of the United States. I ignored my dreams, as I preferred to travel to "wilder" spaces. I blush as I write this. How my thinking has changed from a few years ago. Now I imagine all spaces as sacred, with secrets and ancient magic.

This has been a year of transformation. Shedding so many skins.

Undoing, unlearning. Coming closer to my essence. It is also the year the volcano island dreams became more vivid. I continue thinking of this mysterious lush, volcanic land that would visit me under the blanket of darkness and was now with me during the day. Beckoning. And then the dreams became even more intense with visions of a fierce lava goddess.

Pele is awe inspiring, with flowing hair and blazing eyes as she emerges up and out of a volcano. Her hair is often ablaze, consumed in fire as she calmly looks on, her eyes penetrating, calling me forward. Come to me. Come to me. Come to me. I am ready to answer the call, landing on her volcanic soil. This place of my dreams feels familiar, known. My ancient soul has been here before. The energy is magnetic, hypnotic, and palpable at the Halemaumau crater of Mount Kilauea, the home of Goddess Pele on Hawaii's Big Island. I can feel my heart thumping, my breath catching in my throat, my palms sweating as I face the home of Pele in deep reverence and respect.

I whisper out to her, "Here I am. I have come to you. Why have you called me?" There are many vents of smoke and steam, her lava bubbling four feet under the crust of her crater home. I feel another emotion bubbling up alongside the reverence. It feels quite confusing and disorienting. Out of place. The opposite of the deep reverence I feel for Goddess Pele.

I'm not able to identify it at first, as it feels so out of place in my state of curiosity, reverence, and respect. It bubbles and boils up to the surface. Closing my eyes, I allow myself to feel into it. My breath catches in my throat. I am experiencing agitation. Annoyance. It's anger—the emotion that usually has me at the extremes, unable to flow in a healthy way, either ending in suppression or, at the other end of the pendulum, with an explosion or eruption, leaking all over everyone around me. At first, my reaction is to push it back down, swaying toward suppression. I'm in the middle of paying homage to an ancient Hawaiian deity. I am feeling anger, annoyance, frustration, irritation, agitation, and now, at the heels, waves of guilt and shame for having these intense feelings in a sacred place. My internal critic chimes in, "What is wrong with you? Why do you have to ruin everything?"

I could feel myself shrinking. Wanting to disappear and hide away, to be like the smoke that dissipates from the volcano's vents around me. But being in the presence of an active volcano, smoke swirling in the area, black lands all around, something begins shifting within me. I deeply sigh, exhaling the breath I didn't realize I was holding in. I acknowledge my old friend. Anger is here with me. This is what it feels like to be rage-y and furious. In this shift of acknowledgment, anger's accompanying friends, shame and guilt, begin to fall away. That's weird. They love staying for the party.

I continue to feel into and honor anger. I can't remember a time feeling so liberated in my anger. Feeling so *normal* in my anger. It feels like freedom. It's okay to be angry. I allow myself to stand straight before Goddess Pele and feel through my anger. The anger feels like she wants to move, and my body definitely wants to move. I start to shake. A rhythmic pounding of my heels on the earth, my arms following along. Shaking is one of my practices for feeling and moving through strong emotions. And so, I shake before the volcano. Allowing myself to be with the emotion. To feel the anger, to allow it to ripple through as I shake and shake. I ignore the looks and how others perceive me, closing my eyes. I shake and shake until it feels complete. I then stand tall and wide before the volcano, allowing the mixed feelings of relief and freedom to wash over me. Such sweetness. Such expansiveness. I breathe in gratitude for the shift and can feel the power of my energy. I feel the blood coursing through my body. I'm alive. I'm free. I'm powerful.

At that moment, I understand. I have been initiated by Goddess Pele to embrace the inner fire, what I have always seen as my darkness. To allow my shadow self to be acknowledged, honored, and expressed. I have feared and despised the hot, fiery emotion of anger in me for much of my life. My weakness. My toxic trait. Seeing this as something to fully control—overcome, bury, hide, or unleash all over the people I care most about in the world. Always the extremes. No middle path. Goddess Pele opened my eyes. She gave me permission to be my full, authentic self. She showed me that I no longer need to fear or hide my anger. It is an emotion that has a story to tell, a truth to share. The ultimate alchemizer.

Pele has more lessons in store during this trip around Big Island. More than 50 kilometers away from her home on Mount Kilauea, in and around the village of Pahoa, I see the destruction and devastation of the eruptions, fissures, and lava flows of the volcanoes. It is jarring to see the once lush, fertile rainforest lands covered in black, barren volcanic rock. For miles upon miles as far as the eye can see. It feels like a visual representation of what unconscious, blind, unhinged anger and rage look like. Yes. I'm being shown how damaging and harmful out-of-control anger can be, where aggression and hostility reign. The sacred inner fire, the ultimate alchemizer, is nowhere to be seen.

And then I'm shown another lens. I witness areas that are completely surrounded by the barren lava rock and yet are somehow untouched by the lava. As if Pele controlled the flow of lava, willing it to bend and move to her will. I witness a home surrounded 365 degrees with volcanic rock, as far as the eye can see, while both its front and back-yards and the home itself are cocooned in safety and protection. Hmm. Another lesson: if the direction of a raging river of lava can be swayed and guided, my currents of anger can surely be directed as well. I am giddy with excitement and curiosity. Since childhood, I have always connected with nature and better understood my life in the context of what happens in nature. And now Goddess Pele is speaking my language, showing what is possible in nature, which means it is possible in my own life as well. The lesson lands deeply within me. I am walking on smooth black volcanic rock. I bend down and place my hands on the rock. Sending my deep gratitude to Goddess Pele and the universe for sharing wisdom and this life lesson in a way that speaks to my soul. I bow my head in deep reverence and, hands still on the lava rock, ask Goddess Pele for help in integrating this lesson in my life.

I move on and find it is time for Pele to share another lesson in expanding how I interact with the fiery emotion of anger. I visit the shores of Big Island and learn that as the lava meets the sea, it cools and extends the shore further and further out, creating brand-new land. More than seventy new acres of land in about five years. It was astonishing and awe inspiring standing upon new land that had not been there a few short years ago. The lava has the ability to create new lands. These same hot and fiery flows that ravage and destroy fertile land also have in them the potential to birth something incredible, life giving.

I am being shown both the destructive and transformative power of anger, rage, and fury. This powerful life force energy, if honored, allowed to lead and expressed with intention, has the potential to channel and ignite something beautiful, creative, new, and life giving.

The experience on Big Island cracked my heart wide open. Another shedding of how I had been taught to treat my anger and the stories around what it meant about me. I see now this experience with Goddess Pele and witnessing the lava flows was opening me up for the next unraveling and shedding that came a month later.

My birthday.

Each year, the day of my solar return is ushered in with angst, frustration, and annoyance. In the past, the lead-up usually leaves a wake of tension, arguments, and hurt feelings. I can see now, I often pick fights with my nearest and dearest. I was not actually aware of this pattern until this year. An unconscious pattern that has repeated for decades. Until I became curious about the anger-like feelings cropping up in me. It was always about the other—something said, not said, done, not done. With a heart cracked wide open, it is much easier to ask questions, to get curious, to become aware of the patterns, to feel through and ask these emotions what they are sharing with me, what they have been trying to share with me for a long time.

Loneliness. Grief. Sorrow.

I am floored. I had spent most of the year before unfurling layers of sadness and grief. And now it was showing up again. It was still there? This feels exhausting. It had been intense enough facing, processing, and integrating the lessons from the year before. It almost felt like being back at square one, another beginning. My critical mind screamed that all this healing was never ending. It just brought me back to the same place. My journey from living in my mind, a place of reason, control, and judgment to living in my heartspace, a place of intuition, surrender and infinite possibility, allowed for the gentle and compassionate observation of my mind, and the settling back into my heartspace.

Okay. Coming back into my heartspace. This was another missing piece of my life puzzle. A piece I was ready to uncover and unravel. It would not be showing up at this time in my reality if I was not ready for it. It was a crucial piece to my growth and life evolution. I felt this deeply in my bones. Connecting with my higher self, I asked for guidance on learning more about the grief and sadness that was somehow connected to my birthday. Over the past year, I have been taking myself (and others) into the Akashic Records, the realm of soul imprints where each soul's journey—past, present and future—is recorded. It would be through the Akashic Records that things would be revealed. This gift naturally opened up as I walked the path of my shadow, my light, my self-love, and my coming home to myself.

I was taken to the day of my birth in this lifetime forty-six years ago. My mom had always told me I was born in the midst of a snowstorm. A whiteout kind of day where it's hard to see your hand in front of you, snow whipping about in every direction. I saw the snowstorm; my mom wasn't kidding. I was born in a blizzard. The chaos continued inside the hospital. I'm in one of those newborn beds at the end of my mom's hospital bed. We are pushed up against a wall in a hallway. There is a constant flow of people—doctors, nurses, patients, visitors, paramedics—and noise, so much noise. It looks like I've just been born. I wonder why my mom isn't holding me. I wonder where my dad is. There is a piercing, wailing scream. I look around the hallway, unsure of where it's coming from. I'm taken closer to my newborn self. It's me. I'm screaming at the top of my lungs. I'm red in the face. It looks like I've been crying for some time. I look at my mom. She is looking at the wall, off in a faraway place. Her heart is not with me, here in this chaotic hallway where I've just come into this world. My newborn self senses my mother's distance. This precious baby is scared, disoriented, and alone. Why is no one responding? Despite all the chaos and people, I can't help but ask: Where is everyone? Why am I left all alone with no one to answer my wails?

I feel the depth of this baby's sadness and confusion. My own sadness and confusion. It's the same feeling that I now recognize has always been under the front of angst, annoyance, and anger around my birthday. I have felt loneliness, aloneness, sadness, and grief from the day of my birth. This has been with me from the very beginning of this life. My heart cracks open wider. Tears stream down my face as I witness the sorrow and anguish of this little being.

I see my mom stirring; she stops a doctor who is passing by in the hallway. She asks him if her baby is all right: Why is she crying so much? I feel so confused watching the scene; why wouldn't my mom just pick me up and hold me? The wails are suddenly replaced by loud sucks. The newborn has found her thumb. My mom falls back into bed and turns toward the wall again, and the doctor goes along his way. It hits me; I learned self-reliance from day one. The corridors are now filled with my loud thumb-sucking. My adult self feels an overflowing love and compassion for this little baby. After some time, my dad enters the hallway. My mom has fallen asleep; she does not see him. I watch as he approaches the newborn, and then as he begins to back away and turns on his heel down the hallway. The baby is awake; she has seen him and felt the energy shift when he looked upon her. Her eyes are big and sad. My adult self begins to sob louder. The baby continues loudly sucking her thumb.

I am the second girl in my family. Born at a time when girls are not welcomed or wanted. Female infanticide, the act of killing newborn girls based on their gender, has been rampant for several generations in my ancestral land, Panjab, India. I muse about my own life. Blessed with two miracle daughters who came into the world welcomed with pure gratitude, reverence, and delight. While my husband and I celebrated our family's journey, more than a decade-long fertility journey wrought with much pain, anguish, and heartbreak, I remember the murmurings I heard from some others: "Too bad I have another girl." "I can start trying for a third, for a boy." "It's not too late." An entrenched patriarchy whose insidious reach is deep, wide, and long.

I leave the scene of the day of my birth, that bustling, chaotic hallway, with a little baby in the middle of it all, this new life alone, unseen, unloved. A few days later, I am having chai with my mom in her apartment. I was born on my mom's birthday. We will be celebrating our joint birthday soon, in a few days. I bring up the day I was born, my mom's birthday, and I ask her to tell me more. She starts with the snowstorm. And then she shares more than she ever has before. Because of the storm, the hospital was overflowing, and she gave birth to me in a room, but then I immediately had to be put in the hallway. She tells me my older sister was in another hospital on the day I was born, strapped to a bed, upside down. A new treatment for hip dysplasia. My mom recounts her heart being torn of just having a new baby while her other baby is alone, undergoing a difficult treatment. She wanted my older sister to be at the hospital, to meet me, her little sister. She tells me I cried a lot when I was born, but then I found my thumb and it was the loudest suck anyone in the hospital had ever heard. Doctors and nurses would stop to see who was making all the noise. I ask why she didn't pick me up if I was crying. "It wasn't done in those days. The doctor didn't want me to pick you up. Thinking back, I can't believe I just listened." I hug my mom, hard.

Later that night, I sat with all this new information. My mom was trying her best. My dad was trying his best. Culture, society, ancestral wounds—we all are imprinted with their conditioning and programming. I know they love me deeply, and it's my responsibility to shed another layer of skin that no longer serves my life. I begin the process of reparenting my newborn self. Meeting my baby self in my heart center, gently holding her and rocking her. Showering her with all the love and safety she sought on that first day of life. Letting her know she is welcome, she is wanted, she is loved. I continue this practice to this day, now part of my daily self-care ritual. Allowing her to finally feel safe in this body, safe in this world.

My birthday came and it went. My family had a beautiful celebration for me, filled with so much love, affection, and warmth. My loving husband. My two precious baby girls. My own baby self was in my arms the whole time, being rocked and feeling all the love around us. My dad, who is now one of my guiding ancestors, was at the gathering as well. I felt his loving presence giving that little baby in my arms so much love, affection, and attention.

Opening to my anger, honoring my anger, getting curious about it on that fateful day before the great lava goddess, allowed for a deep discovery of self and a subconscious story that I was holding onto from the day of my birth to emerge. As I process and integrate the many truths of anger, I can feel its alchemizing power working within me. Forgiveness, compassion, and peace rise to the surface. I have a feeling future birthdays will have a much less negative charge, perhaps even a spark of deep joy and serenity.

Chapter FIVE

Awakening the Body-Mind

Lindsay Lesage

It takes awareness and education to know what works for your own nervous-system health and wellness. It's up to you to find your secret sauce.

@_lindsaylesage

Lindsay Lesage

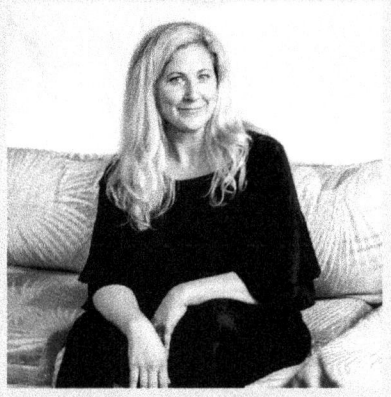

Lindsay Lesage is a wife and mom of two. She lives by the shores of Georgian Bay, Ontario. She and her family love cycling and skiing and playing together by the Bay. She is passionate about helping people change the way that they think in order to change the way that they live. As a wellness coach and positive neuroplasticity teacher, Lindsay is passionate about sharing knowledge and guidance to improve quality of life and increase energy, mental wellness, and joy!

INSTAGRAM @_lindsaylesage

For Quinne and Henry

Awakening the Body-Mind

Over the last decade I've taken countless courses and workshops and read an inordinate number of books about the body and the mind. I would even go so far as to say that my knowledge in this area is extensive. And yet to this day I would say that attuning the body to the mind and the mind to the body is still my biggest work in progress. I'm slowly coming to terms with the fact that this journey is ongoing and that you can't just learn something, do it once, and solve the issue when it comes to the mind–body connection. I roll my eyes when people say things like "that's why it's a practice," yet that is the absolute most hardcore truth I've come to learn.

In 2014 I became a certified yoga teacher because I had found myself struggling to deal with the stress of the school-teaching world that I had recently entered. I was shocked at how stressful I found teaching, yet I should have seen clearly that it wasn't the end path for me.

In 2010 I was in teacher's college and experienced for the first time what I would later learn was called "moral injury." In essence, moral injury is when you see a large defamation or injustice to what you feel are morals that should be upheld. The theories, values, and dreamy teachings of my professors about what education should and could be sparsely matched the classroom reality. Where we were taught that we are the vehicles for change and for the empowerment of students, the reality was that we as teachers are often counselors, parents, mediators, nutritionists, and sometimes (yes, I cringe to say it) babysitters.

Without going into too much detail about those first few years as a teacher, let me just say that I was an excellent student while growing up. I would listen, obey, and strive to earn the approval of my teachers. And I honestly didn't think that there were students who didn't. I must have had blinders on as a kid or was just too busy working hard at toning my perfectionistic qualities that I somehow missed the reality of a diverse array of student types. And now, actually being the teacher (you know, "the one in charge"), I thought that my students would do what I had done, which was be respectful and ready to try their best and work as hard as I had as a kid. Looking back on it now, I see what a ding-dong I was and how embarrassingly naive I was about it all.

I began to become extremely tired and exasperated by the teaching job. I felt like I wasn't able to uphold my perfectionistic tendencies and gain what I thought was a successful cohort of students if they weren't able to do the same. It became a deeply personal reflection on my skills and abilities, which I now understand is absolutely bonkers. I was most certainly burning out from caring so much that I worked in the evenings to prepare for the next day's lessons and never had any time to rest, relax, or do the things that really helped me unwind and restore. I was desperate to be the best teacher and that meant having extremely smart, driven, and capable students who would quietly listen and get straight to work and produce. In psychology we call this cognitive dissonance—when you have an idea about how something should be and can't shake it when the result doesn't turn out as such. Deep down, I knew that my students all came from diverse backgrounds, experiences, and socioeconomic statuses, yet I still couldn't part with the perfectionistic piece of myself that wanted them to be more capable. I was doing the best I could, and so were they, but my expectations of myself just weren't matching up, and I was constantly striving to be better and to do more, and I was absolutely exhausted.

This is where the yoga journey came in. I figured I was too young to be this stressed out about teaching and that if I had some skills to help me calm down and chill out, then everything would be much easier. I'd been to a few yoga classes, and I liked the physical challenge and always felt refreshed after Savasana; plus, I figured I'd be toning myself into great bathing-suit shape. This would be perfect, and I would no longer feel stressed and overwhelmed by school and teaching, and I'd look great in leggings. Win-win!

I remember thinking I'd found the simple solution to burnout and being quite proud of myself as I bounced into the first morning class high on an "aren't I so clever" kind of momentum.

I walked into those first few weekends of yoga teacher training just as naively as I had walked into teacher's college. In the first few hours of this training, I was cracked open and crying tears that I didn't even know needed to be released. *What the hell is this?* I thought. *This is crap, I feel like crap, and I'm trying to not feel like crap!* I was pissed that I had made what seemed to be a huge mistake. I just wanted to relax and wear some lululemons, for goodness' sake!

Throughout those first few weekends, I was not happy and thought for sure that I'd made the wrong choice. And so much for looking good in leggings—I'd been emotional eating during all our training breaks. I was pushing my body, my mind, and my emotions way harder and further than I thought I would be. This simple solution was starting to feel convoluted and hard and counterproductive. I honestly contemplated quitting.

But then I remember sitting with our anatomy teacher during one lesson, and she said something along the lines of "the issues are within the tissues." And something clicked. She wasn't referring to the number of tissues I'd gone through crying my eyes out so far into this training, she was referring to us holding our stresses and our emotional and mental issues WITHIN our bodily tissues. All of a sudden I understood what she meant. I understood it all. I understood why I was crying so much and so often during the movement of my body. I understood that this is exactly how I was releasing the issues—by moving them out of me. I later heard other phrases that clicked, like that our shoulders are where we keep our "shoulds." This one resonated big time, as I have always had incredibly rock-hard shoulders and have a hard time not wearing my shoulder blades as earrings.

It was then that I became fascinated with anything related to connecting the body and the mind. My whole life I had been obsessed with psychology and the philosophy of emotions and the mind. I had spent upward of eight years in therapy at this point in my life and nothing had felt better than moving my body and releasing what was being held within. Up until that point I had been living from the neck up. As a very intellectual and academic person, I had never understood or listened to myself from a visceral perspective. I have zero recollection of stopping myself from eating when I felt full as a kid or listening to my body to see what it might've needed. I remember stuffing my face when I had big feelings, and I remember pushing my body so hard to win a race at recess that I would end up having asthma attacks. There was never a happy medium. That all began to change as I deepened my study of yoga.

I became particularly enthralled with Yoga Nidra, which is essentially "body sensing." It really is as simple as bringing your awareness to a body part in space and time and sensing that it exists. You can literally do it anywhere at any time. Try it! Just bring awareness to your toes. Sense them. Move them or not, but just bring your awareness to them. Now bring your awareness to each toe one at a time. Big toe, second toe, third toe, fourth toe, baby toe. There, you just did the basics of Yoga Nidra, or body sensing. There is incredible research by Dr. Richard Miller or iRest Yoga Nidra that shows that this simple awareness of bodily sensations can reduce instances of anxiety and depression, and it has been shown to aid in the management of PTSD.

Fast-forward a few years and I had been teaching school and teaching yoga simultaneously. I had a few regular classes per week and would also host day retreats and workshops. I enjoyed it, and it was a great way to really continue to listen to my body and tune inward. I still found teaching school to be incredibly stressful, and I was continuing to struggle with balancing everything, but at least when I was moving my body and tuning inward, I wasn't so caught up in the perfectionistic perspectives and had a lot more self-compassion.

When my sister was diagnosed with breast cancer in February 2017, we used a LOT of Yoga Nidra to get her through the pain of surgeries, chemotherapy, and radiation. I remember texting her in the middle of the night when she was in the hospital recovering from surgery and I knew she wouldn't be able to sleep. I would walk her through some Yoga Nidra practices, and it would help when the painkillers wouldn't. My sister then became obsessed with the practices of Yoga Nidra and

Restorative, and we would eventually go on to host workshops and retreats together. We were working together on our biggest retreat yet when we were forced to cancel it due to the pandemic in 2020.

Meanwhile, I had fallen out of my own practices and started living back up in my head again. It started with my first pregnancy, as I felt so sick and uncomfortable that any type of movement felt extremely arduous. I look back now and know that I also used my first pregnancy as an excuse to be lazy. I was exhausted from working full time as a teacher, traveling, having a podcast, and teaching yoga on the side, and I had also been at school training to become a psychotherapist. It is clear to me now that I was back in my perfectionistic zone, trying to "do it all" and strive for more. During that first pregnancy, I experienced what I felt was an unprecedented kind of bullying from my dad's girlfriend at the time, something that caused a major splintering of our father–daughter relationship. I felt a ton of feelings coming up from my childhood that I had stuffed deep down. My parents had tried their best with our childhood, but in hindsight, we all see the cracks and where we needed more from them. My parents split up when I was nineteen, and although it was devastating, they remain extremely caring and gracious of one another, and I am very grateful for that. Nevertheless, I had no idea that pregnancy and child rearing would unveil so many deep wounds of the past. No one wrote about that in the baby books. No one spoke about this aspect of becoming a parent in the birthing classes that we took. I felt like, once again, I was naive to the truth of a situation that I thought would be a certain way and took a completely different turn.

When my daughter was born, I transformed from maiden to mother in an embodied way. Our birth story is not untypical where again I thought it was going to go a certain way and it didn't. We ended with an emergency C-section after hours of my pushing. I had never even entertained the idea of a C-section in all the birth prep we had done. After my daughter's birth, I was more connected to my body than ever, yet the messages coming through weren't just the sensation of milk letdowns. Rage, anxiety, and tears all showed up for no reason. I felt like a caged lion and was extremely protective of my daughter. My husband got me a gift of newborn baby photos when my daughter was ten days old, and when the photographer was holding her and trying to bounce her and calm her down because she was screaming, it took everything in my body not to rip my baby out of her arms. I felt like a literal mama bear. I would feel anxiety in my chest if anyone other than my husband was holding her. It carried on for a long time like this, and it was exhausting. A year and a half later I felt like I had just started to get a handle on these mixed-up bodily sensations. It had everything to do with exercise. Because of our birth ordeal, my body took a very long time healing from surgery, and it was hard to move or exercise the way I needed to. However, once I started moving again, everything shifted. This time it was harder movement than yoga, and it was helping tremendously. I was boxing and doing cardio and feeling great; I will even go so far as to say that I was feeling more like myself again. And then we found out that we were expecting our son.

This time around I kept moving for the sheer fact that I had a two-year-old to chase after. I kept doing cardio and going for lots of walks. While they definitely helped my body recover faster from the planned C-section with my son, my mind–body connection went haywire again. Having a C-section means doing very little movement for at least six weeks, which is ridiculously difficult with a toddler running around and a newborn needing tending to. If I'm honest, I didn't transition well at all from one to two children. Perhaps it was another case of how I thought it would be versus the stark reality of how it was. It was the biggest struggle emotionally because I felt like I was always letting one of them down. My daughter was crying because I was feeding the baby, or my son was crying because he needed to be fed while I was trying to pour love and attention into my daughter. Eventually, as my son got older and my body recovered and the snow began to thaw (both in the environment and in what felt like my internal winter), we began getting a handle on it.

But the biggest reason that things shifted was because I began to learn more about the nervous system and the effects of what is called "dysregulation" and "regulation." I had learned about self-regulation as a teacher in terms of teaching this behavioral skill to our students and in reference to students who lacked this behavioral skill. However, I had never heard of regulation and dysregulation in a bodily sense.

Once I learned that our minds follow our bodies and its reactions to the nervous system (fight, flight, or freeze), and that the behaviors are merely a symptom of these reactions, everything clicked. I began to see all the scenarios that I previously explained from a regulated or dysregulated point of view.

In teacher's college and those first few years of teaching, the moral injury and injustices I witnessed caused my nervous system to dysregulate. When I was a young teacher and had students throwing chairs at me and swearing at me, my nervous system went into complete stress and dysregulation. When my body went through pregnancy, labor, and surgery, my hormones and the physiological changes caused my nervous system to dysregulate. When I brought home a newborn to join our two-year-old, and both demanded my attention after I had gone through major surgery and sleeplessness, it caused my nervous system to dysregulate.

The patterns are so clear now and learning this felt like a major weight lifted from my psyche. For the longest time I thought that I was too sensitive and put too much pressure on myself and that it was all due to behaviors and emotions that I couldn't seem to get a handle on.

Once I realized that these were in fact somatic reactions that were trying to get out via behaviors, I had a newfound awareness that allowed me to work through anxious feelings, intrusive thoughts, and behavioral patterns that no longer served me. It takes practice to stay in that place of awareness, but the more I do it, the more I am now able to name what was happening and move my body in order to metabolize the stress and regulate my felt sensations or emotional reactions.

Nervous-system regulation can come in many forms. It can be through yoga and meditation, it can be through supplements and a deep look into your dietary lifestyle, it can come through sobriety, it can come through exercise and a proper sleep. The truth is that there is no one-size-fits-all and that it takes awareness and education to know what works for your own nervous-system health and wellness. It's up to you to find your secret sauce. I truly believe that mental wellness is like a puzzle: there are many different pieces, and everyone's picture of it looks different.

Chapter SIX

Homecoming: Connecting the Dots to Return to Yourself

Anita Rombough

We spend our lives looking outside ourselves for belonging, acceptance, worth, and love when it is inside us all along.

@anitarombough

Anita Rombough

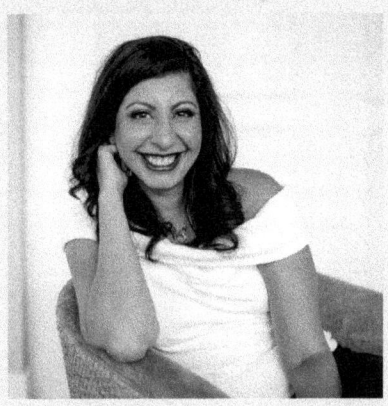

Anita Rombough is a soul strategist, success coach, inspirational speaker, and host of the wildly popular *Anita Chat* podcast. As a gentle yet bold change agent, she helps fellow big-hearted dreamers align with their soul or "sole" purpose to achieve their version of success. Above all, Anita is passionate about amplifying the potential, fulfillment, and impact of herself and others. In her downtime, you'll find Anita creating memories with her family, traveling, in nature, on her yoga mat, or relaxing at home with a good book, or her tarot cards.

INSTAGRAM @anitarombough

To my parents, my husband Greg, and to my biggest blessings and cheerleaders, Bennett and Jiya, for your unwavering love and support.
And to all of you who are brave enough to dream big, honor your truth, and step out of your comfort zone to come home to yourself.

Homecoming: Connecting the Dots to Return to Yourself

What do you want?

I could feel my heart beating in my chest. Unexpectedly out of the blue, a manager asked me the very question that I had been thinking about nonstop in my head.

My purpose, my *why*, my creative spark felt like it was getting dimmer with each passing day. I didn't know where it'd gone, and I didn't know how to make it come back. And as I walked around, going through the motions and feeling like an impostor, I felt like I had been exposed.

Quick, what do I want?

My answer was rapid, composed, natural, and true. I wanted growth and challenge. I wanted to create impact. I wanted my work to mean something, and most of all, I wanted it to feel fulfilling. Was it lying by omission to mention that this role was no longer checking off all those boxes? Sure, it supported a great mission. I was proud of our vision and my personal contribution. I knew I showed up day after day and gave my all to this role. But I was increasingly feeling like the work and mission weren't being set up for success. While I knew it was time to leave, it was difficult to reconcile a steady, healthy paycheck, work–life balance, a generous vacation bank, and a pension. People would kill for this job. Why was I dying to get out of it? More importantly, what was next? Deep down, I knew I was meant for more. I just didn't know what more was.

Ever since I was a little kid, I've been consumed by finding my purpose and my home in this world. A place where I belong, feel whole, and am accepted. As a kid, I led a very lonely life. I was bullied relentlessly. Peppered into a sea of white upper-middle class as one of a handful of "ethnic" kids throughout all my school years, I didn't have fancy things, name-brand clothes, or fancy rides. As an only child of my immigrant Indian parents, I came from very humble beginnings but had big dreams.

Finding safety, security, and belonging as a kid meant playing small, trying to go unnoticed on the playground. At home, it meant being the dutiful Indian daughter who did well academically and made her parents proud. It meant being responsible, reliable, and perfect. Back then, I found peace, comfort, and companionship in the pages of books, writing in my journal, and in my spiritual practice. Of my own accord, I had set up an altar in my room and would spend hours a day in deep prayer and ritual. Around the age of ten, I taught myself to meditate with the help of a cassette tape bought at an ashram gift shop. I remember fishing for the sky-blue cassette cover with a magnolia tree illustration in my collection of homemade top-forty mixed tapes and putting it into my black cylindrical two-door boombox. When following the instructions of Swami Rama, our beloved guru, I remember wondering if I was meditating correctly, since this was far before the time of YouTube and Google. Nevertheless, I committed to the practice regularly, feeling a newfound sense of peace and calm in my anxious and worried mind.

I was also incredibly intuitive from a young age. I remember going into the variety store with my dad at around age five and adamantly insisting that he purchase a specific scratch lottery ticket. I'll never forget the look of surprise and delight on his face when that ticket was a big winner. Elated, he held me up in the air as if I were a trophy. My gifts of inexplicable "knowings" and ability to manifest things at whim as a child continued. By age twelve, I was accompanying my aunt to yoga classes every week. To this day, I'm grateful to her for introducing me to yoga. My mat has also become my happy spot.

As a high achiever and people pleaser, I went on to complete three university degrees with distinctions such as making the dean's honor lists and being the class president. My first degree was in psychology with a minor in biology. I was fascinated by how our mind works and how it is shaped by our beliefs. While pursuing that degree I discovered and fell in love with occupational therapy (OT), a health-care profession that considers the many facets of a whole person rather than looking at a person as a physical body or medical diagnosis. Despite falling in love with the philosophy of OT, fairly soon into the degree I "knew" that it wasn't it for me. Still, I enjoyed the learning and committed to extracting as much from the opportunity as I could before moving on to something else. About ten years later into my career, when I owned my practice, I "knew" it was time for another change.

I traded in my first grown-up apartment in the city and my newly achieved debt-free student loan status to move back into my parents' basement in my late twenties, this time to pursue my master of business administration (MBA). This would be my first big "pivot," returning to school as a "mature" student. Unlike with the other degrees, this time around I only took courses that I was interested in. I didn't come into the program with any preconceived agenda or plan for specialty. This was such different energy from the prior degrees where everything had been focused on earning the degree, not learning from the degree. At the end of the program, I graduated with distinction as a strategic marketing major. I also met Greg—my future husband and father of my two precious children—in Accounting 101.

I found myself back in health care after graduating, this time working on setting policies and best practices and doing large-scale transformative work. I loved being at the helm of creating change and impact for the greater good. It was deeply gratifying until, out of the blue and close to a decade later, I felt like I had outgrown the place. When I looked around, I didn't want my boss's job, or my boss's boss's job. Though this workplace was big, I couldn't see a position that sparked my excitement. Once again, I felt like I didn't belong, and it wasn't where I was meant to be anymore. Juggling feelings of stuckness and restlessness during the midst of the pandemic, I felt the Universe leading me down a different path.

About a year and a half earlier, I'd had this inner knowing as an intuitive that I needed to write a book. Aside from a childhood love of writing in journals, I had no topic in mind and no know-how. As a result, I kept pushing this nudge out of the way until one day it became a deafening scream. Unable to ignore my intuition anymore, I sat down with my journal and asked the Universe for help. I specifically asked if this was meant for me to give me the people, resources, tools, and opportunities to make this happen. At that precise moment, when I put the period on the sentence, my phone chimed so loud that it caused me to jump off my seat. It was alerting me to an email that invited me to participate in a free writers' challenge with a major publishing house.

Sign from the Universe noted.

As I delved deeper into writing, I started having thoughts of coaching and picked up courses and training to support me. My wish was to impact as many people as possible, and as fast as possible. We were in the midst of the pandemic, and many people were struggling, looking for deeper meaning and purpose, and I "knew" I could help them through my past experiences, education, intuitive gifts, and track record as a successful therapist.

Locked down, working remotely, "momming" so hard, and now writing and studying, I had a lot on the go, but that spark of excitement was back. One day in my prayers, I said, "If this is the work I'm meant to do, I would really appreciate having more time and money to spend on it." About six months later, I was part of a corporate restructuring with all the time and a healthy severance package to support me. Once again, the Universe delivered!

Unlike the planned life transitions before, this unplanned transformation brought with it some complicated emotions. I felt free! I felt free to veer off the traditional path that I was on before and to chart my own course. On some level, I also felt shame. I always excelled at school and in my career. Although it was a business decision, and others were also uprooted, it felt immensely personal. After spending a decade of my life with an organization and largely tying my identity to my work, it felt like my second family had shut me out. On that note, how would my parents react? I'd spent my life wanting to make them proud. And let's not forget fear and doubt. Who did I think I was to try this? What would happen if it didn't work out? I had a family to think about now. In looking around at my friends, I didn't know many that had made as many career changes as I had. How come I didn't have this figured out already? Was this truly a sign from the Universe to delve into entrepreneurship? It certainly was risky.

Despite the uncertainty that surrounded me, there was also much clarity. Like a game of Connect the Dots, in hindsight, the Universe had perfectly orchestrated each and every single event to set me up for success now. Growing up, I'd faced significant challenges, but they made me resilient and instilled a strong belief in myself. Personally and professionally, I proved that I could overcome any obstacle with my determination and strong work ethic. Through my lifelong connection to the Universe and my spiritual toolbox, I discovered my higher self, which enabled me to connect with others on a deeper level. My expertise in mindset methods allowed me to understand why people behave the way they do, while my experience as a therapist taught me to appreciate and support the multifaceted complexity of those around me. Through my work, I helped countless people achieve goals that were meaningful to them. My strategic leadership contributed to large-scale transformations in health care with far-reaching implications. As an MBA graduate, I even had the marketing know-how to promote myself. It seemed obvious that the next dot was to put all this together and serve others as a soul strategist and success coach. A few years into this work, it still feels aligned and perfect for this evolution of me.

After finally giving myself permission to break away from tradition and explore new, uncharted territory, my life has evolved into a consciously curated journey that brings together all parts of me. This journey has led me to a place of peace, deep purpose, and inexplicable joy. Today, I'm able to use my expertise and unique gifts to help others connect with their true selves, achieve their most meaningful successes, and experience the fulfillment they desire beyond their wildest dreams. As an impact-driven change agent, I'm grateful to support others through my coaching, podcast *Anita CHAT*, and my writing. It is humbling to think that the quiet, unseen girl who once felt worthless and trapped by scarcity has become a confident, empowering, and charismatic leader who shares her voice and truth with people all over the world. I never imagined that my "big dream" would be to help others live theirs. Not a day goes by when I am not filled with gratitude and honor for carrying out this deeply fulfilling purpose.

As a fellow traveler on the life journey, I don't know where this dot will lead, but I can share what I've learned based on my journey thus far:

- We are always home. We spend our lives looking outside ourselves for belonging, acceptance, worth, and love when it is inside us all along. As a part of this process, we try on different personas to see what feels good and what others validate. We find home when we are unapologetically and authentically ourselves. This is also an extremely vulnerable and courageous thing for us to do. Do it anyway.
- The cliché "home is where the heart is" is a truth bomb. Most of us, while navigating our lives, choose our heads over our hearts, but when we truly tap into the wisdom of our emotions and the vibration of love, we discover our inner GPS system that guides us home to us. Let your feelings be your compass.
- Everything that has happened in your life has unfolded exactly the way it was meant to for your highest and best good. Trust, even when it feels hard.
- You are always changing. Each day brings new revelations, new

evolutions, new challenges, new strengths, new wounds, and new triggers. Allow things to be revealed on their own timeline. This is part of the journey that will get you to the next dot.

- Our lives are our own biggest mystery, and we are the star detectives piecing all the universal breadcrumbs together. Not only are we the detectives solving the mystery, we are also the narrators of the story. Our beliefs, whether empowering or limiting, create the overarching framework for the narrative. You decide your story. Choose a good one.

So now, my friend, it's time to ask you the same question that was asked of me. What do YOU want?

What would you want if there were no limitations or obstacles in your path or if you knew you couldn't fail? That inner knowing is your truth. When you lean into and trust your truth, all the right tools, resources, and opportunities will be placed on your path to support your purpose. If you are questioning whether this is as good as it gets, if you feel like you are settling or aren't excited or scared, you aren't playing BIG enough. Those dreams you have are yours and only yours for a reason. Welcome home, my friend.

Chapter SEVEN

Whispers of Growth

Jessica Brasier

It is in the "in-between" where joy is found. Not in the "will do" or "did" but the DOING . . . that is what really creates the magic.

@lovinglifeessentials

Jessica Brasier

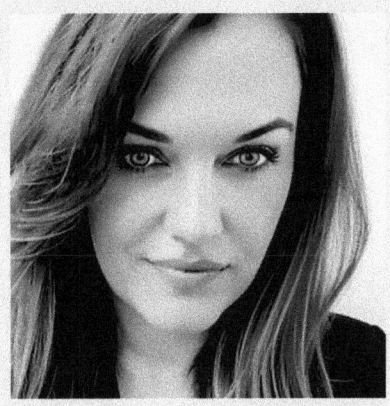

Jessica Brasier lives in New England with her husband and five children. She is a wellness advocate and someone who trusts herself to ask questions when she seeks to understand, who stands up when something doesn't add up, who is always wanting to learn to do better, and who will always speak what's on her heart. Jessica will set out alone on a path if that is what she so chooses. Additionally, she knows others will understand her, not by her words but her actions. She hopes to empower you to do the same.

INSTAGRAM @lovinglifeessentials

This chapter is affectionately dedicated to my husband and my children whose interest in this, as in all my ventures, is never less than my own.

Whispers of Growth

I often hold the hand of my inner self and hear the whispers of growth, the warnings and rewards of all that I have learned and experienced. I hope to guide her through what is to come. I think back to choices I made and don't even recognize versions of myself that look and sound the same, but then there is a shift from judgment to compassion. "I did my best with what I had. And I am still trying, still healing, and always still learning." It is through this lens and lesson that I have found the passion to share it with others.

We can't forget to be most kind to every version we have ever been that has gotten us to where we are today. This gratitude anchors us in a way that reminds us that the purest form of love has to come from within. It is from that place that we can come home—to make room and make way for growth and expansion.

Practicing this opens us up to a whole new way of being—being more present and accepting of what is happening in the world around us while also making way for awareness and openness to our inner world. I found that by doing this, we can have more moment-to-moment present experiences and a welcomed sense of peace from the hustle and overwhelm of a systematic life we created in a fogged tunnel vision of pursuit. Those whispers we hear come in loud now, right and wrong, yes and no, right or left, and become so clear that when we listen to them, we begin to experience a deeper connection to our bodies, and we become more aware of the emotional and instinctual alignment of our lives. We are also learning to love ourselves with kindness and curiosity. We begin to see and offer grace for the habits we have chosen and changed and how we think and relate to new life experiences, often persistent but also, at times, temporary.

I am a wife, mother, entrepreneur, and advocate. So many roles and titles, but the truth is, I cannot be any of them (at least not well) without knowing that me being me is not what I do but who I am. And in my experience, who I am changes from time to time, and should, to further my evolution. Doing so with love creates so much joy, and the type of joy that has the mind, body, and soul not just balanced but zinging in the best way!

There will be many adventures in life that plant, grow, and bloom you to a new radiant blossom . . . over and over again. We rarely see the in-between messy twists and turns; we only know where we are and where we want to end up. It is my belief that it is in that "in-between" where joy is found. Not in the "will do" or "did" but the DOING . . . that is what really creates the magic.

This has been the case for me for years. I have spent most of my adult life caring for people. Hell, if I look back even further in time to when I was a child and the oldest of three, I remember being the neighborhood babysitter. If there was a child, elderly relative, or pet in the area, I was often hired, sacrificing my nights and weekends to tending to others. And I loved every minute of it! I have been assuming responsibility for others' care for as long as I can remember, something that has brought me purpose and joy for "helping" in any way I can, especially when it is received in gratitude. I can think back to a time in my adolescence when this looked like volunteer work with non-English speaking immigrants and providing support services for poverty- and addiction-based community care and companionship centers.

As I moved into adulthood, I continued seeking ways to "provide support" through medical care, behavioral/home health, and volunteering. I was driven and eager to please, all things that would be the desire behind the sacrifice I'd continue to give others despite myself, which would prove to mean nothing compared to the simple quiet gratitude of health and happiness. These roles brought me great joy and purpose, experience, and a ton of education to share, but ultimately, they all required me to put others before myself. They took me far from "home" because of the imbalance between sacrifice and fulfillment. When virtue signaling is disguised as self-love, things are bound to get a little messy.

My inner shift began in 2009 when my youngest daughter, at age four, had a fourteen-foot fall, and in a miracle, had zero signs of injury. A few months later, however, she started to have "spells" that we eventually had diagnosed as epilepsy, which we were told she was sure to outgrow. Sure enough, a few years and a few staring spells later, my daughter was a well-adjusted healthy and happy little girl at age seven.

In 2010 my husband and I moved our family to a neighboring state, chasing what we thought would be a safe, exciting, and better financial opportunity. My husband quickly excelled and was promoted as the youngest and best master of his trade in not one state but three, reaching a position we believed would create a lifelong career. I settled into managing our home and started to feel comfortable enough to let that ambitious nudge blossom again. I enrolled in school and took a job where I was once again the helper, creating value in ease of service for others.

In 2013 our daughter's epilepsy was once again active, so I withdrew from school to be available to her, which was something that felt purposeful. She needed me, and I needed to know she would be okay. Life changed in time. School for her became my time to continue "working" as if I still believed there was value in overextending myself. I heard whispers of "be still"—whispers I have heard many times in my life, but just like every other time, I ignored them. A few months later I had the unexpected happy yet life-altering news that we were pregnant again, this time with our fourth child. It was a complete surprise and a blessing I will always be grateful for. I let my then-boss know I wouldn't return after maternity leave, as my new child would need me to be present.

The whispers continued: "be still." In some act of rebellion, I took the next few promotions, and when the time came for maternity leave, I walked away with a smile on my face and a sadness in my heart. What should have felt like accomplishment felt again like sacrifice. I adjusted as usual to the new life of a mother of four, and I liked it—loved it even. Actually, I let myself fall in love with creating a home with our children and the life my husband and I created. We were thriving, and it felt safe. We talked of purchasing a new home and creating a lifelong future in this new place.

When our newest son was months old, my husband underwent surgery for an injury that would end his career. Now we would have to really get creative because we'd created a life around an income we no longer were earning. My husband suggested moving back to our hometown. He often missed the simple life we had left behind years before. To him, this was a "sign" or perfect timing to make the move. I was angry. I had a full-on tantrum. I was not ready to leave the life we created just as it seemed to be starting, and when you add in the postpartum hormones, it made for a wild time in our home.

"Be still." This time I heard it. I knew what was being asked of me, and I didn't see a different way. I used the remainder of our savings to move and purchase the closeout of a local consignment shop. I was going to open it locally wherever we moved, thinking self-employment would give me the freedom to care for my ill daughter, injured husband, and new baby. I leaned into trust and moved our family back to an area that, in my mind, would offer zero growth but would give my husband peace of mind. He'd stay home with our children, and I'd support us financially. If I felt like another sacrifice, I started to see a pattern.

We settled into what we call our "struggle years," remodeling his sister's basement with rooms enough to fit our family. I opened my boutique and went to work, hoping to save enough to buy a home ourselves. But due to the weak economy in our rural area, I was forced to close my store. I was heartbroken. Why did things align so perfectly but then fall flat? I scooped myself up and took a "normal" desk job: regular pay, proof of income, consistent history—all things mortgage companies love. I began to have debilitating panic attacks and anxiety, but I couldn't place why, because to me, as nutty as it sounds, I had no reason to be stressed. I thought I was in complete gratitude; instead, I was coping with what is known as toxic positivity—the pressure to only display positive emotions while suppressing any negative emotions, feelings, reactions, or experiences. This invalidates human experience and can lead to trauma, isolation, and unhealthy coping mechanisms.

I would not surrender to it. Instead of ignoring the whispers this time, I would ask why, what, and how. Perhaps I was finally determined to find the path to wellness. I put one foot in front of the other.

In the spring of 2018, we bought our home, an accomplishment that had us over the moon. Synchronicities of familiar alignment showed up to let us know we were in the right place. A few months after my daughter had her first of many true Grand Mal seizures and an ambulance ride to the emergency room, we were told that it was likely the seizures would continue and maybe even get worse. Once again "be still" had me feeling the pull to be home to not miss a moment. I worried and thought, *What if the next time I lose her?* I needed to find a way to create an income within the parameters of comfort.

It was almost as if as soon as the thought would come up that I should expand my wings a bit, something else would happen to ground me back to family. My husband suffered a complication with his injury, paralyzing him for days. Having my daughter's seizure and my husband's complication happen in tandem and having three other kids to care for sent me to my knees. I once again started asking questions and discerning the answer I felt, then moved in little baby steps, as I was now almost scared to really move until there was an astounding "YES." Then, three years later, with my daughter's seizures "managed," the Covid pandemic began. I felt a pull to listen even closer and seek clarity. With so much misinformation and fear-based energy swirling about, I felt obligated and honored to have the voice and experience to educate and empower others.

Following conversations about wanting to make an impact in collaboration with a few other professionals in my area, I opted into participating in a collaborative wellness center, and once again, I really started to adore the life I was creating, this time with purpose and freedom to navigate growth as an entrepreneur as well as flexibility for family.

I heard it again: "Be still." It began feeling more like a warning to hold on tight because life was about to give a lesson learned the hard way, but with purpose.

Within four months, my oldest daughter, still in high school, a runaway who also happened to be a stranger from thousands of miles away, showed up pregnant on our doorstep in need of healing and a home. And once again, after years of quiet, my daughter's epilepsy became active again, this time with frequent episodes of seizure activity that would leave her absent and more in need of care than ever before. For days I laid by her side and asked God to bring her back, to rest her mind, and to give her back a quality of life I could support her through.

With great misalignment and a priority to focus on healing in the home, I withdrew. It broke my heart to think of leaving something I once again created in love. I was building something of value, something that I believed at the time was the way to make a difference. I didn't see at the time that the value I was creating was the path back home to myself, and it was getting easier and easier with each challenge and each opportunity I was given to choose me above all else. To lean into the whispers and grow.

I suffered burnout, self-abandonment, and disassociation without having the skills for or understanding of how to climb out of such an automated darkness. Time began to stand still, and progression was lost. Limiting beliefs and toxic self-talk of "how can I help someone when I can't help myself" became my inner dialogue, which created a cycle of nervous-system deregulation.

Learning that there is, in fact, a difference between assuming responsibility for something that is not mine to carry and something that I can contribute to in support and love was the piece I needed to start again. But it was not an aha moment; it came in more of a culmination of these whispers of love and guidance, becoming the freeing statement to re-light the path home. It took me a year of being planted in the heavy but nurturing soil of my life before I would be cracked open, reaching for the sun.

Once I felt relief, I knew helping others find relief was something that needed to be shared and modeled. It starts with becoming aware of the things that need to shift. I call this "getting curious" about where we get to (yes, I say "get to") do the work. Because the work that will come from this space of curiosity will change our lives for the better. Messy sure, a stretched discomfort without a doubt, and at times with our mind turning on us in search of the comfort of "safety," but it will also crack us open to grow and bloom in a way that radiates joy and purpose. It will become a familiar feeling of growth, and when seen in gratitude rather than fear, the entire process is welcomed in light. It's magical.

This self-awareness also creates a sweet spot of exploration for how to have stronger and healthier habits and to practice and have relationships with ourselves, as well as with each other. Our intuition, our bodies, our emotions, our health, our finances, the spiritual realm, and all aspects of our life and the ripples that come from this self-awareness will start you on your journey of coming home to yourself.

We often forget how to love ourselves through becoming, through growing. The truth is, life often makes us tough through experiences that aim to teach. Our nervous system regulates in a way to protect, and as much as that is a blessing, it can feel restrictive and even fear inducing, creating limiting beliefs that often are responsible for stopping us before we even get started. It's the fight, flight, freeze, or fawn state. I know them well.

We have all been there, right? I find peace in knowing they are here to keep us safe, so they will not go away but rather pop up in a way to lovingly remind us to pay attention and reach for the tools we need to support and balance.

When we all find ourselves in this cycle, it's in the HOW that we can nurture ourselves through this process. There are many ways to do this to work with your unique needs, but a good place to start is to be AWARE, to thank the belief or feeling, then let it go in love. This may sound or look like "thank you, fear/limitation, for showing up to keep me safe. I am so grateful for your love. I no longer need this protection. I will release you now."

You will start to feel yourself getting lighter without the weight of these limitations pressing down on you. Now you have space to create new positive beliefs.

With awareness and without limitations, you have created a clean slate to now rebuild your life coming from your new perspective of love. There is a sense of excitement and joy that comes from this place of newness and freshness; it's a honeymoon stage for all the treasured parts of yourself. It's in this space that you will take on new habits and create a day by design that turns into a life you have only up until now been dreaming about.

I suggest getting really clear and protective over this time. Soak it up for all its worth and anchor it in so that you can revisit it, because like a real-life honeymoon, it will end and shift, offering us a new perspective, deep intimacy, and treasured gratitude for the next step.

It's at this time we start to cycle back around and DARE to do it all over again in order to find our way home, even sometimes in the dark: with Desire (What do we want?), Awareness (Why do we want it?), and Reflection (Wow, can we do it). Then you Execute (With action, what are the steps to get there?). DARE can be applied to all areas and aspects of your life when you are feeling that it's time to pivot. These are the fundamental building blocks to come back home to yourself.

There are many modalities to support you as you shift and become aware of what is needed to evolve, from talk therapy, frequency support, plant medicine, body movement, nutrition, rest, detoxification, to others. My life changed for the better when I began to love myself each day with one or many of these. I created a lifestyle around nourishing my mind and body, and in return, they loved me back. It's a powerful thing when you create a home within yourself and then light the way to always find your way back. Be rooted so deep that flying feels free.

So today, from a place of joy and peace, I move in and out of desire despite the limits that try to consume. I check in with myself often to offer support and care as and how I need. I now have self-trust, self-worth, and healthy boundaries, all of which allow me to do what gives me purpose: be a resource of experience and education in a way that honors who I am and who I will continue to become.

Life will ebb and flow and experiences will come in fast and sometimes linger. Knowing who you are and what you want and how to get there is the easy part; it is in the brave steps and the choices of becoming that you will illuminate your own growth and path home.

Chapter EIGHT

Remember Who You Are

Apryl Jennings

Waking up is a mix of remembering who you are and being willing to forget who you aren't.

@apryljennings

Apryl Jennings

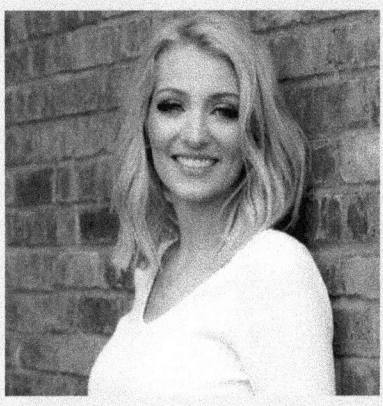

Apryl Jennings was the number one international leader for a global company when she left her job to pursue her soul's purpose—serving those who are looking to move from religion to spirituality. Apryl is an avid studier of esoteric work, which she translates into simple and usable wisdom for everyday life. She strongly believes that people are born to serve, and that life has prepared each of us for it in a unique way. A mom to four littles, she is most proud of moving away from fear-based religion to seeking truth for herself and her family.

INSTAGRAM @apryljennings

To my husband, who's walking it out with me.

Remember Who You Are

Have you ever made a huge move that no one else could understand?

I left home at seventeen years old with a backpack and ten dollars to my name. I was running away to live with my soldier boyfriend who had just returned home from a tour in Afghanistan. I grew up in an old-school Baptist home, and so did Drew, this boyfriend, who is now my husband of thirteen years and the daddy to my four babies. I was seventeen years old but much older mentally. Children raised in religion often grow up young. We grow up aware of the world on a larger scale. Mortality and morality are daily topics. It is a way of life that is unique. So much of my upbringing was beautiful. I have many moments of joy. I didn't plan to leave the church or to leave my family and then THIS! This moment in time came up, and I had to go. I was being pulled and guided by an inner voice.

Drew and I were given the options of "break up" or "break up." Drew had left the church and become part of the "world"; thus, he was not allowed to date me. I hadn't had many crushes on boys growing up, but with Drew it was different. I remember the moment I met him. I've come to realize that we remember the moment we meet someone when they are a key player in our life plan. It's like this little soul spark goes off. Something in me said GO! HIM! He's part of your story.

On this fall day, at seventeen years old, I got into a taxi and left home. I followed my heart. It was the saddest day of my life. I chose my heart, and my world chose the church. I thought that leaving my family that day was the part that made me so unbelievably sad, but it wasn't. It was the belief I accepted that day that brought the sadness. In that moment I accepted the agreement that leaving church meant leaving God. I accepted the label of "black sheep." I accepted that I was a failure in the eyes of the church, and since the church was my symbol of God here on earth, I was also a failure in the eyes of God. We make agreements without consciously being aware of them.

I tried to go back to church so many times, but I couldn't. Every time I went, it felt gross in my body. I was being given a very clear "NO, you cannot go back to this way of life," but I missed God so much. I just wanted to go home, and I had no way there. I lived like this for a decade—not sure where I fit in and feeling completely lost. I had barred the door to religion closed and tried to rebuild my life from scratch. I wouldn't talk about or process my childhood. If Drew brought up the church or the Bible, I walked away.

I felt I had been royally screwed by life in one specific area, and I was mad about it. Most people are supported by family when they leave home. They build on the education they have been working on their whole life. They have connections they've made through their family and maybe even some help with secondary education. I had to build from zero. I had spent almost eighteen years learning about a Bible and religion I didn't want to touch with a ten-foot pole. I couldn't understand how this was fair.

I ran for success, trying to find some feeling of worth. I knew something was missing, and I couldn't seem to find it. When you are driving and you see someone running on the sidewalk, it is quite easy to know if they are running for the joy of running or if they are searching for something they lost. The woman who is searching is frantic and committed. She will go through the rough terrain or run in the dark. She knows she's lost something. She knows there is something to be found. She will run harder and faster than someone who is merely running just to run. She will run until she finds what she's lost or until she collapses. I collapsed. I thought I was searching for success, but when I found it, I still felt empty. I still hadn't grasped what I was searching for, so I kept running. I found more success, more influence, more stage time, and I still wasn't home. It was maddening. I just couldn't seem to get there. There was a door in front of me that I had barred closed, and it seemed so unrelated to how I was feeling. It was the door to my childhood. I knew I couldn't go back to that religion, but I couldn't figure out how to get back to God.

When I collapsed from the decade of searching, I found myself at a Tony Robbins's event called Unleash the Power Within. I had attended it for business reasons. What I found was a spiritual awakening. A moment of grace I can't explain but will forever be grateful for. It was the last moments of the last day, and I had fully committed to the whole forty-eight hours. The days were long. I saw a look on Tony Robbins's face that spoke to my soul. There weren't words. Spirit speaks to us in knowings, and we translate them into words. Tony wasn't even talking. The music was playing loudly, and he was looking around with tears streaming down his face as he saw the thousands of people on the screens dancing and celebrating our four days together. My soul screamed, "That! I want what he has!" What I was seeing was Peace, Love, Joy. I was seeing Pure Spirit.

I knew his beliefs were different from what I was raised with, and yet he had peace. I had never seen this look of serenity and peace on anyone's face while I was growing up. Those people who had claimed the angle on God did not have this overwhelming peace; they didn't have Spirit. That was it! It sounds so simple, but one look was all it took, and I was AWAKE! I opened to the idea of unbarring the door to God. I was about to march back to my childhood and take my divinity back. Maybe God was something other than what I had always been told. I had hope for the first time in a very long time. I realized that maybe, just maybe, there was more to this story.

That little opening of my heart was all it took for the Universe to blow up my life. I didn't realize it yet, but I had just woken up from soul sleep. **I had just left the first phase of life**. I was about to find my purpose. I went on to let go of a business I had spent years building. I dove into reading hundreds of spiritual books and divine texts, studying work from many masters. It was an obsession, and I LOVED it! Books that I needed found me. Strangers handed me books. People I didn't even know who were watching my journey offered connections that furthered my growth. Mentors seemed to pop out of thin air. I was divinely guided as we always are when we are brave enough to step on the way. I felt I was finally on the path that led home.

What I came to discover through this seeking was a unique teaching that has helped so many to finally understand their life and realize their soul's purpose.

There are two phases of life:

There is the first phase when we are born into earth school and are in soul sleep. We agreed to this before we came here. Nearly 100 percent of who we are is invisible. This part of us knew we would be born sleeping. We knew we would be born into the "hell" portion of our story. Hell means confusion. And it is awfully confusing and hard to make sense of life when you are sleeping. You actually can't quite make sense of it. It's like asking someone, "What are you dreaming and what does it mean?" while they are still sleeping. They can't answer you. In the dream, the monster is still scary. In the dream, you don't have the awareness yet that this monster was only placed on your path for you to become a champion. In the dream, there is so much fear.

So many religions have tried to explain this part with words like soul sleep, hell, illusion, and confusion. It doesn't matter what we call it, but it is extremely powerful to know that it is going on. In the Western world, we have taken this phase of confusion and placed it in the afterlife, which ironically, has caused confusion. It isn't in the afterlife: it is here and now, and it is a state of mind. It is something we agree to before we ever enter this school. It also means it isn't an accident, and you aren't lost or in need of saving. You are walking out phase one of a two-part agreement.

Because we aren't aware of this agreement, most never wake up and become the true version of themselves. We all live through this phase of life. This stage is hard. This is where you question why you were even born. You feel you are at a disadvantage when you look at others. Life doesn't quite make sense yet. You may feel lost, and this is also why the term "lost soul" is often used for this phase.

GOOD NEWS: You are right where you need to be, and the best part of your life hasn't even happened yet.

I learned this teaching from a rabbi, David Cooper, in his book *The Mystical Kabbalah*, and it has always stuck with me:

"Think of yourself like a house. When you see a house, you are instinctually aware of the fact that before this house appeared on the spot, there was an architect with a vision. There were blueprints drawn up. There was a team assembled and a plan put into place for a time and location to make this dream a physical reality."

There is a master architect and a plan for you. You aren't here by coincidence. Thinking you are is what has caused pain. Wayne Dyer said, "There are no coincidences." None! Your infinite, all-knowing self chose to be you. This house you see is the holder, the vessel for your eternal, pure self, the holder for who you actually are. You aren't the house, you are what lives within it. You are the formless part.

I know you know this deep down. I'll prove it. Imagine with me for a second (and I pray this never happens to you), but imagine that you are sitting next to a close friend and she slumps over without warning and passes away. What would you do? You would say her name. Then you would scream her name. You would shake her shoulders and yell, "Are you okay? Are you there?" Why are you screaming her name if you can see her? What is it that's gone that you are searching for? You are screaming for her consciousness to respond to you. What you are frantically screaming for is the invisible part of her.

Ponder this: You are formless and eternal.

Let's dive in deeper. You choose the perfect playground for your soul's development. Then it happens. You come forth into time and space and the "forgetting" takes place. Here you are. Born into a name that comes with a whole prewritten identity. Seeing yourself as the name on your birth certificate. Fallen completely and deeply into the sleep of the soul. You identify with all the roles written into your story to fully gain the experience. You are the sister, the daughter, the mother.

You are feeling it all and gathering what you will need to know for the second half of your life. Every main lesson you want to learn is attached to a bond that you can't get away from. It is attached to people who have titles like mom, dad, uncle, grandparent, best friend. These are the people we call soul pods. You come forward together.

At this point in the game, you've completely forgotten that you are an infinite being. You've forgotten that you are pure LOVE, and everything is always okay. You are playing the game you signed up for, and you're playing hard! You aren't doomed or lost or wretched. You're simply doing what you signed up for: gathering experiences for the second half of life—for heaven.

You're walking it out, sole on the ground, while gathering experience for the soul. Earth school is where the sole and the soul work together. You are enrolled in earth school, and every school comes with a curriculum. This is the part of the teaching where people usually want to slap me. They say, "Apryl, I would never choose this life." And I agree; same here. If I had chosen my life, it would be a lot different. You and I, the very dialed in version of us, the names on our birth certificates, wouldn't choose this. But here is the key part: that isn't the part of you who chose it. It is the "you" that goes with you through every lifetime that lines it up. While you still think this "house" is all there is to you, you will be in pain. You will be in confusion. You are fighting life. I would like to help you move into accepting life. Until we realize that we chose this life, we can't accept it and zoom out. We must get to the point where we can look at our life and say, "I accept that I chose this. Show me why."

When I realized an infinite being signed me up to be Apryl, I started to look at my arena differently. I stopped fighting it and started working with it. I started to surrender. I didn't find my purpose until I accepted my life. I finally said, "If you chose my life, then show me why you would choose the upbringing I had. Show me why and I will listen."

My biggest question? "Why would I choose a religious upbringing if I was never going to use it?" It wasn't that my childhood was bad, it was that it seemed irrelevant to the lifestyle I was living now. I didn't see how it fit into my story. In fact, I was convinced that it didn't.

What part of your life do you question the most? What doesn't seem to suit you? Where in your story do you say, "I don't know why this happened?" or "I will never use this part of my story."

There is a common belief that children until the age of eight are just walking around downloading their parents' beliefs. An identity is being formed within them. A "normal" is being decided. We knew this fact was how the human worked before agreeing to be poured into one. Think on this: you knew the influence your parents would have on you, so it is not a coincidence.

I hope at this phase you are realizing that absolutely nothing about you is "irrelevant" to your story. If you are struggling to find your unique purpose, I can guarantee you that you have some parts of your life barred up.

The second phase:

Phase two is the reason you were born. The Biblical scriptures say, "The second man that cometh is the Christ." Some call this second phase "the Christed Self." Tony Robbins calls it "the Giant within." Some simply call it "AWAKE." I call it returning home.

When I finally opened the door to my religious past and processed it all, I realized that my purpose is to free people who were raised with religion. I was born to remind people that they are God in a body, and no one can take their divinity from them. I realized quite quickly that the part of my life I had questioned the hardest was placed there as preparation. It was never where I was meant to stay. This was why I felt it wasn't my choice to leave, I was being told GO! The preparation phase was done. I wasn't meant to stick around and marry a preacher boy. I had to get out or I would miss an important intersection in time.

Once I was awake, I could explain it all so clearly! My soul came with a mission and moments of grace in place to serve as alarm clocks. I chose to listen to my alarm clock. Where I started off my life was the opposite of my destination. It wouldn't be much of a journey if there was no destination. We are in a school of polarity. I had to walk my message from hell to heaven. When we stay in pain, we are missing out on our true life. You were never meant to live and die and stay sleeping.

Pain turns into power once we can give it meaning.

I now spend my time helping people who were raised with religion become free.

Those eighteen years of religious upbringing that I didn't want to touch with a ten-foot pole have come in awfully handy. I have had so many people come to me who are riddled in fear from old religious beliefs, and I can walk them to peace every single time because I know the way out of their specific hell. Place me in that hell and I'll become free every damn time because I know it!

A tour guide wouldn't be very successful if they had never been to the area before. To lead others out you first need to know the way. If I hadn't lived the first phase of my life, I wouldn't be able to serve in my purpose. The moment I stopped running from being ME, unbarred the door to my past and looked around, the whole puzzle came together. I understood that Life was never screwing me over; Life had filled my toolbox to overflowing with resources. The only piece missing was ME being willing to be ME!

Now, I wouldn't change ANYTHING about how I was raised. To teach it you must know it, and to know it, you must have lived it. There is something that happens when you live an experience. It is recorded in your soul's memory, and now when you speak on it, you are powerful. If you are ignoring parts of your story, you are missing part of your power. I've had some clients tell me they are worried others have the same truth to share as they do. Here's the thing: no one can take your message because what makes your message powerful isn't the truth you are sharing. Let's be honest. Anyone could Google some good truths and stand on stage or post on Facebook. What makes your message powerful is the road you walked on to find that truth. It's in the blending of sole and soul experiences that we become powerful. People *feel* you more than they hear you. They feel the message behind the words. This is why when someone is sharing their *true* story, we cry. We feel their soul mixed into their voice. Your unique story matters! Your voice becomes powerful when you mix it with your own experience.

So many of us left our story back in childhood. That thing you are hiding; that thing you refuse to talk about; that thing you question with all your being—that thing is ready to be transmuted from metal to gold. It is through sharing your story that you will heal it. Until you do this healing, you carry the lower frequency of your message within your body. You carry the "first phase frequency." Forgiveness means exchange. When you forgive your past, whether self or others and probably both, you will exchange your old frequency for the healed version of you. There is a second version of you that you were actually born to be. She isn't owned by her story, she is owning her story. When I stopped running from my story, I became free.

Your message is hidden right in your childhood. You need to go back and find that gold. You need to get to the point where you can ask, "Why did I choose this specific life experience?" and be open to the answer. Then get a bowl of popcorn and dig in!

The first half of my life, the downloading of the limiting beliefs, the identifying with the name on my birth certificate, it all created a story and an avatar. Someone I wasn't, but someone I agreed to be for the experience. We aren't truly ourselves until we think for ourselves and our "first man" is compiled of everything we've ever been taught. When you wake up, you become a free thinker. You question what is and isn't you anymore. This is why others often get upset with you. This is a process you must go through. This is the step between phase one and phase two that is called "dying to self."

So many of the greats spoke on this. They said, "Be no one but yourself"; "Imitation is suicide"; "To thine own self be true." Why did they find it so important to warn us about this? Like anytime you give a warning, it is because not listening is dangerous. Because they knew the importance of being YOU! Not the *you* in the confusion, but the *you* who knows who the fuck you are. The *you* who woke up and realized life filled your toolbox to overflowing for the true life you were born for. You are equipped for your perfect self-expression.

Waking up is a mix of remembering who you are and being willing to forget who you aren't.

We are all here to walk ourselves home. How could we walk home if we didn't start far away from it?!

We are all here to walk from hell to heaven. If you're brave enough to go on the journey, maybe you'll come out on fire and light the way for others.

Chapter NINE

Finding Light

Ashley Anne

The future is bright.
Darkness doesn't live here
anymore.

@_ashannne

Ashley Anne

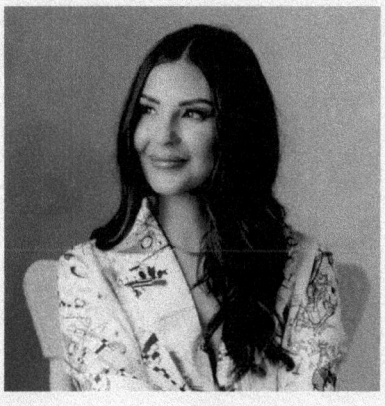

Ashley Anne saw the ins and outs of darkness several times within her first twenty-nine years of life. It wasn't until she was faced with the life-changing struggle of becoming a chronic pain warrior that she truly understood how dark and deep the hole of depression can get. She shares her own experiences to show people that you cannot only keep your head above water but also learn to swim great lengths. Ashley Anne is the founder of Real-Life-Shit Features, a clothing brand dedicated to mental health awareness. She uses this platform to feature warriors of all kinds who have gone through their own version of real-life shit. Ashley Anne believes that we are stronger together, which is why her first of many books to come was a collaborative effort with other strong and courageous women. The power of reading helped Ashley Anne live the twenty-nine years that were written *for* her; the power of writing will help her conquer the next thirty-plus years that will be written *by* her. Everyone is invited to join the story, as it will help seek out resilience within darkness.

INSTAGRAM @_ashannne

To my two father figures. I truly believe I wouldn't have reached this place in my career without the lessons that they left me with, and this dedication is my thank you.

Finding Light

What's in Your Trunk?

- My cosmetics and self-care items (a suitcase on its own)
- Another for shoes
- One large luggage bag filled with clothes rolled tight like pitas for maximum space
- All of Daisy-Dog's essentials
- Blankets and pillows
- Summer floaties

That's what was in my trunk on August 4, 2022, when I left my apartment, my long-term boyfriend Dylan, and my other dog and my cat to travel to the East Coast of Canada to spend time with my brothers. When I left my home in the small town of Peterborough, Ontario, almost two hours northeast of Toronto, I had no date of return, nor would I provide one. When asked if I was coming back, my response was "it's 50/50." I had the contents of my trunk, Daisy-Dog riding shotgun like the queen she is, and in those moments, that was all I needed to survive.

I knew my returning was even less likely than the 50/50 chance I had provided, but this takeoff was already so painful for EVERYONE: not just for Dylan and me—our families felt this pain as well, as we had truly all become one. Our friends felt this motion too, but for different reasons. I wasn't going on a vacation; it was a quest: a quest to fill in the gaps of my life and repair the cracks of my heart and provide me with another to find value within myself.

At the time, I had been having serious health complications for nine months. My symptoms consisted of sharp and burning shock-like feelings in all my joints that sent waves of pain through my entire body. The pain felt like a full-body lightning strike, and it was partnered with a stiffness so intense that it caused mobility issues. This pain started only in the left side of my jaw . . . what a strange place for pain, right? With the location being so unusual, I was first diagnosed with three ear infections, receiving a different prescription for each one. From there, I had my throat checked, which also came back fine. I even had X-rays done of my teeth, which guess what? Also came back fine!

The pain and stiffness never stopped. The symptoms became more severe and traveled down the left side of my body. The right side was compromised shortly after. This was one of the scariest times of my entire life. And I must point out, I was well supported! I had one of the best support systems you could ask for, but even still, it was traumatic in many ways.

I had difficulty walking and needed help most of the time, either with the use of a cane or by lovely people taking me by the arm. I'm sure you can imagine that being assisted to the door of the hospital by your eighty-year-old nanny could be a bit of a wake-up call to your situation. Climbing stairs was next to impossible without assistance, and once, I fell up the stairs, causing such a severe break to my hand that it required surgery. My boyfriend had to wash my hair for me during this time, bless his heart.

I went through months of testing—multiple MRIs, CAT scans, trips to the doctor's office or Emergency Department (ED)—and more trips to the lab for bloodwork than I could ever begin to count. And even still, I wasn't getting much in the way of answers. Each doctor I saw tried different medications to make me as comfortable as possible. The first thing I was offered was narcotics: Percocet, Morphine, Oxycodone, etc. Not only did I feel extremely uncomfortable with medication of this variety, but they also did nothing for my pain. I felt dizzy and even further cloudiness in my head, but my severe pain points remained the same.

One day I went to the ED in tears, begging that they try something other than a narcotic. Truthfully, I wasn't even really sure what else there would be without a diagnosis, which was very similar to what I was told medically, but they still tried! I began treatment-based medications for nerve pain and inflammation, which led to a breakthrough in my pain levels. *Thank goodness.* Shortly after, my family doctor added a medication into my routine that helped with the stiffness and referred me to the Toronto Pain Clinic for further testing.

I didn't wait for the appointment in Toronto. I should have, but the wait for answers had already felt like an eternity and was slowly eating away at my soul. As soon as my mobility improved and my pain was somewhat manageable, I jumped in my car and headed to the East Coast to visit my three brothers, unsure if I would ever return to my life.

I've already said that I had the best support system that anyone could ask for during this time: I had a long-term relationship with my best friend of twenty years, three pets, and a beautiful place to call home, so you're probably wondering how I could have just left everyone who loved and supported me. It's a fair question that I have asked myself several times, and I can provide you with a long list of answers:

I was unhappy that I'd existed within a friend group that was toxic for much longer than I should have. I had a strong desire to find like-minded individuals instead.

I was unhappy in Peterborough. I knew I would be, but I'd moved there anyway, for someone else.

I was unhappy that I'd allowed myself to crumble within the pressures of my life.

I was unhappy with my constant pain and immobility.

I was unhappy that I'd lost my previous career, which I loved, due to health complications. My having a career of any kind felt far out of reach during this time.

I was unhappy that I was no longer able to keep up with my loved ones or participate in the activities that I was used to doing.

I was unhappy with the overwhelming number of judgments that had been coming my way regarding my health, from doctors, certain family members, friends, and even strangers.

I was unhappy that I'd felt like a genuine burden to all the people who loved me.

But most of all, I was unhappy with *me*. My unhappy state, combined with the traumatic memories of Peterborough that still haunt me in my sleep to this day, all became too much. I was saddened to depths I had never experienced before: I was sleeping all day, plus I had uncontrollable mood swings and emotions that came through as tears, and frustrations that came out as screams. In my opinion, I had become incredibly hard to be around. When I look within the intention of this behavior, my belief is that I was trying to push my loved ones away, not to hurt them, but to help them. What I might do to myself in this state felt terrifying and unpredictable. I no longer felt like I was contributing to society, to my ride-or-die relationships, or to the promised commitments within my life. I saw no worth in my presence without my usual abilities, which ultimately led me to the "what's the point?!" feeling within my own existence.

But even with that lost sense of self, I wanted to find the point. I didn't want to continue feeling like a burden to people who would NEVER let me struggle. I wanted to try making my way back into the working world and without all the previous judgments that put cracks in my soul. My career and my contribution to society are two things that have always meant a great deal to me. I was not about to give up easily, nor was I prepared to do it in the same location where I relived my worst memories. My surroundings lacked motivation, the people in my life had gone through enough, and I felt far too intimidated to show my new ability, or lack thereof, to the only people I had ever known. It was at this moment that I filled my trunk and drove to Dieppe, New Brunswick, all in one go!

In that fourteen-hour drive, I had never felt so free. I was driving long distance for the first time in nine months. The weather was beautiful, the car windows were down, and the breeze flowing through my hair felt like it was taking the pressure off my shoulders and replacing it with the feeling of fluffy clouds. The sunshine beating down brought out the light from within me that had been replaced with shadows for the better part of a year. I was exploring areas that I had never been before, which filled my spirit with wonder and imagination for the future.

I had never done a road trip by myself, although I wasn't alone because I had Daisy-Dog. She'd automatically begun acting like a service dog when my health issues started. She'd never left my side. The more severe the pain, the closer she was to me, and she would even bark at people when she thought I needed something. My having her there gave me and everyone in my life a strong sense of security. During the road trip, us stopping along the way for dog walks and nourishment breaks was the best bonding time we'd ever had. Providing care to her in such unique circumstances began to reengage my sense of purpose.

My stepfather was also on my mind for the entire road trip, providing me with an additional layer of security. I was raised by my stepfather, and we had a unique father–daughter relationship for the twenty-five years we were blessed with having. He wasn't always easy to be around, and neither was I, but we never gave up on each other. We argued when we needed to keep one another on the straight and narrow. My stepfather struggled tremendously with mental health concerns of different kinds. I struggled with anxiety and depression throughout my teen years. I also worked full time during my high school education. I had a desire for nice things and the need to buy them for myself. Whenever I needed a reminder that I could take on the world while dominating work and school, my stepfather was always there to fill my cup with drive (or Molson Canadian), and I was always there to remind him that just because he went through hell, he was so far from evil. His heart was filled with a certain generosity that not many possessed. It was like he was in a constant fight between the angel and the devil, and it devastates me to say that the devil won the day he took his own life in 2019.

This loss left me with an overwhelming feeling of guilt. I felt like I didn't do enough, like I should have been there at that moment, and despite my best efforts, like he didn't know how much he meant to me. I regularly need to find forgiveness within myself for this, and I used the drive he left me with to make him proud of the woman I am.

Shortly after his passing, I saw a medium and requested a message from him. I was absolutely shocked by the results. Everything that was provided to me by the medium made so much sense and was so personal. One of the messages that came through was that my step-father was always with me in the car. This resonated with me deeply, considering he was always on me for my heavy foot, even though my need for speed totally came from him. Thus, before I'd left for the East Coast, I found one of my stepfather's antique CP Rail keys that he was given as a tribute to his service there, and I hung it on the mirror in my car. I knew that he was watching over me, and not just in the car, but also on the quest to find myself.

When I'd been in Peterborough, my stepfather was all I could think about, and it wasn't in a healthy way. It was in a level of guilt that could take down the strongest of soldiers. I wanted to see him in any way I could, and considering how dark I was feeling at the time, that scared me. The combination of depression, my feelings of guilt, and the strong desire to crack a cold one with my old man had me thinking that leaving this world the same way he did could honor him in some way. But his voice screamed from every vessel in my body: "Don't you dare give up!"

He left this world because he thought it would be a better place without him; in his eyes, he gave me a better life. I will never agree, nor will I ever fully forgive myself, but I will absolutely NOT waste this gift. His last gift wasn't of a material nature, it was the gift of my fight for my future.

As I drove out of Ontario, my guilt shifted to unconditional love.

I remembered the woman he wanted me to be: pain-free, motivated, strong, hardworking, and protected. With my health concerns, some of these felt impossible to conquer, but there was no highway I wouldn't speed down in order to fulfill his dream of my future. In his honor, I would find pride within myself again.

As I entered the tenth hour of driving, further traumas continued to process through my mind and transition into fluffy clouds. I had a large division on one side of my family due to childhood sexual assault, and I was beginning to want a relationship with them. I was a girl in this trauma, and I needed to find answers as a woman. I knew some of these relatives were wholehearted people. As far as anyone I was unsure of, I had the confidence within my healing to put myself on the line with the hope to complete my family for both myself and my brother, Andrew.

Andrew is two years older, and between us being close in age and always having to work so hard at our relationship, we are incredibly close. We didn't have to work so hard because we didn't get along, it was because we *barely* got to live together as we grew up. The distance never stopped us, and I've recently learned yet again that it never will. We would visit one another, wherever we were living at the time. And we used FaceTime daily, texted nonstop, and even planned activities with friends at the same location in order to see each other and to merge our friend groups. Although this was misguided, at the time we felt our friends were all we had, thus making it important for us to know who the other had for support.

Andrew has been in a polyamorous relationship with Kyle and Randy for ten years now. They resided together in Peterborough for six years before moving to the East Coast. During this time, their home became my safe place. We saw each other nearly every day, and they provided me with some of the most heartfelt gestures I've ever known. During this time, I went from having one brother to having three, and I needed that safe place, now more than ever.

It was 6:30 a.m. when I arrived at their home. Daisy and I snuggled in the car until Andrew realized we were there and opened the door. I should have been ready for bed after that fourteen-hour drive, but there was no way I could sleep. My excitement to be with them beamed from the core of my heart. It was an anxiety-free kind of excitement that felt new . . . like a new beginning . . . and just like that, I knew I was staying.

Andrew, Kyle, and Randy welcomed me with open arms, and I felt so at home, even while living out of a suitcase, which spoke loudly to me. My relatives were sad to know I was far from them, but they were happy to know I was with Andrew. The hardest part was telling Dylan that I was not coming back. Before our relationship, we were close friends for twenty years. When we took a chance on becoming more, we both found such security and genuine happiness within our relationship that we had started to question if it even existed. But it did, and we knew it.

At the time I left, our relationship had been scraped over rocks. We both had people who never supported our relationship, we took a lot of hits, and me trying to push him away probably would have been too much for most, but not for Dylan. He understood how lost I was, he knew that I was spiraling, and if he had to, he would travel to the ends of the earth to catch me as I fell. It's a loyalty that I have never known yet will never forget. As Dylan said goodbye to his friends and family and shipped all our belongings out east to come join me, our love and loyalty reached a level of invincibility. We spent the summer finding ourselves as a couple and as individuals. We traveled, we communicated, and we grew on levels that paved our future.

With the support of Dylan and my brothers, I reached out to my dad's side of the family. This was such an important part in my quest for a whole heart and understanding of myself. He and his family loved me like no time had gone by. We all really needed the strength that their love contained, but we were denied time once again. My father passed away on February 28, 2023. He was waiting for a heart transplant when his health made a drastic turn for the worse. Offering him comfort was all we could do, but you could still see him in pain that nobody deserved. His time came far too soon, but he took it with bravery and courage. In the time that we did have, I learned a lot about our similarities, filled in blanks from the past, and formed relationships that will always keep his memory alive and well.

This sudden loss, combined with the inability to make it to Ontario in time to see him, was scary for us. The thought that we might lose time with our other relatives, from all sides of both families, was unbearable. Our desire for family and my need for Ontario health care now have us returning, and I have the ultimate peace with that decision. I found my independence, made sense of my past, and gained vision for the future.

As we pack our belongings and fill our trunks, I feel so thankful for my brothers and all the long heart-to-hearts we had. They gave me strength and helped me simplify things to find myself, one beautiful step across the beach at a time. As the stack of boxes gets higher, I think about the new heights Dylan and I have found within our relationship. We are concrete, unstoppable, and engaged. As I picture the drive back to Ontario, I know my heart will grow in size for each kilometer traveled closer to our families.

And in the vision of my return, I'm filled with a love I've never known, wisdom that changed me, and a whole sense of myself. I found my light and remembered my contributions to my ride-or-die relationships, to society, and to the commitments within my life. My relationship with Andrew could never be tarnished, as space is all we've ever known, and love is all we've ever had. The relationships in Ontario require more time, nurturing, and support right now, so that is where we will go. Some of them are new relationships, planted like seeds into the earth and in need of water to thrive, and my cup is full. Some relationships are with our angels above who are always guiding us through life. Others are right here in front of us, and we would like a hug from each of you to be a short car ride away. No matter where we are, our loved ones have a permanent spot in both of our hearts: past, present, and future.

The future is bright. Darkness doesn't live here anymore.

Chapter TEN

The Broken and the Beautiful

Chernell Bartholomew

Our body is our one true home, and this journey of becoming is what makes our stories unique.

@chernell.energycoach

Chernell Bartholomew

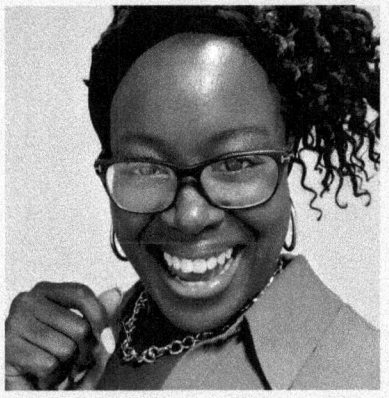

Chernell Bartholomew is a girl mom of three, a certified health coach, a personal trainer, a published author, and an award-winning registered massage therapist. She is living the life she envisioned and helps women capture their vision of health and live it fully. She is passionate about helping women who are on the verge of burnout put themselves first so they can discover their energy, confidence, and power without deprivation or extremes. She is a lover of all things energy, kickboxing, good food, and '90s' R&B.

INSTAGRAM @chernell.energycoach

Dedicated to the ones who feel like they are on the brink of burnout but have a deep knowing that there has to be something more.

The Broken and the Beautiful

As the sun rose, I was about to board a plane to a foreign country with a group of women I barely knew. It was January 2020, and I had been invited on the trip by my business coach who I'd met years earlier, just as I was exploring the idea of building a wellness business. I was a registered massage therapist (RMT) and trainer and wanted to coach women and moms, and this coach had created an amazing online community of moms in business that showed me it was possible to build a business and be a great parent along the way.

We were going to Panama. It was to be a dream vacation filled with personal development, relaxation, and time to focus on my big goals. It had taken me months to finally say yes, even though I'd always dreamed of traveling to beautiful locations for business. I remember talking about it with such excitement and then a bit of hesitation because I was afraid of not feeling good enough while surrounded by these women I admire. I thought I was out of place, that I wasn't at the same level in life or in business as they were. I hesitated because I thought that what I had to say wouldn't be valuable, that I didn't have anything to offer. You know when someone sees something great or special in you, but you can't see it? That's where I was. I thought of myself as good in most things but not great at anything. I had learned through a challenging relationship with my dad that I was supposed to be seen and not heard. That if my opinion was different, it would lead to an argument. That no matter what I did, it wouldn't be the right thing. I never felt like I was enough, and this feeling led me to make decisions in life that kept me small, that were not aligned with my true purpose. Even now I sometimes second-guess going after the big goals that sit with me, and I have to actively quiet the mean voice inside.

So, I faded into life and became the good girl who didn't want confrontation, the one who kept everyone happy but dimmed her own light. Over the years, from within myself and from society, I had learned to quiet and distrust my voice, my intuition, and my body.

I wish I could go back and tell my younger self that you don't have to be perfect, that you're allowed to make mistakes and relearn. You don't have to be tall and skinny; you are allowed to take up space. You can be loud and opinionated. Your pains and fears are valid, but they don't need to hold you back. We are all struggling with the same things. Some just learn to mask it or move through the pain, doubt, and hesitation faster. Rest but never quit, take care of you first, and all else will follow. Build a team of supporters, mentors, and people who test your views and challenge you to grow and those who bring intention, fun, and peace into your space. Say yes to your dreams.

Saying yes to that trip was a big step for me. It started to build back that muscle of trusting myself. It gave me six days of no kids and no cooking, just space and time to dream about what I wanted, who I wanted to be, and what I wanted to accomplish in this lifetime. I gave myself permission to sit at the table. I couldn't quite put my finger on it, but the energy of taking that chance on myself expanded my world.

Doing yoga, standing barefoot with my toes in the sand on the beach in warrior pose, listening to the sounds of the waves rolling in and out, gazing into the blue sky that seemed to stretch on forever, feeling the warmth of the sunrise hitting my face—all experiences I didn't think happened in real life, at least not to a woman like me. But they did, and I truly believe I was meant to be there. On that trip I decided to go after my coaching dream. I decided to lean into personal development. I decided I wanted to be a leader in this wellness space. And I also decided that 2020 would be the year we got pregnant again and completed our family. My energy shifted on that trip.

Your energy is intimately connected to how you experience life. It is connected to who you are and how you show up, your patience, your focus, your vibe. It is the magnificent things you say, do, and create. It is the reason you wake up and feel like you are enough, you have enough, and you can make it through another day. Or your energy is the roadblock that keeps you playing small; it's the reason you curl up and forget your power. It can keep you stagnant or aid your growth. It can be what builds you up and fortifies your spirit, or it can trick you into unknowing.

Understanding and tuning into the knowledge we had as children, that we have choice, we are joyous, our needs and wants matter, can give us power and strength. Energy is everything, and when we forget that we are the creators, the manifestors, the generators, when we get sucked into what the world tells us we should be, should do, should consume, we disconnect from that innate sense of self and pain spreads. We disconnect from our essence and desire to explore, create, and build something meaningful. When we are brave enough to leave our expectations behind, we get to decide how to live our life on purpose.

It's easy to get trapped by the everyday, the obligations, and the comforts, by the overwhelm and the need to blend in, but what I always dreamed of was to stand a little taller, to walk with more self-assuredness, to speak with a steadier tone, and to make an impact on the lives I touch. I wanted to be a voice for the women like me who felt that they needed to do, to try, or to have the latest thing to make themselves look or feel worthy; for the women who didn't look like the standard of beauty or wellness being pushed at us. But I felt I couldn't shout this message because I was still stuck in it myself.

I was stuck being the nice girl, just enough but not too much, smart enough, good enough, but still carrying a deep knowing that I was meant for more. And at the same time, afraid to want more and not wanting the judgment from others or from myself. I carried a feeling that I wanted to blend in and play small, that I was supposed to be complaining with everyone else. But I also wanted them to recognize their worthiness, their capabilities, and their value so that I could choose to recognize my own.

But what about when you don't choose this experience?

It was early 2021, just months after giving birth to my third daughter (like I had decided on in Panama), when I finally climbed into bed for the night. As my husband threw his leg over mine and wrapped his arms around me, he rested his hand on my stomach and I relaxed and smiled. I realized that this confidence, this comfort, this acceptance, and this pride in my body and what it was capable of was different. Just months prior I would have judged myself for not "bouncing back." I would've wiggled my way into a new position or moved his hand, or I would have just cringed and recoiled into myself. That instant reaction of "don't touch me, my body isn't good enough" would have echoed in my head. This once would've been my reaction after having a baby, but it wasn't.

This feeling was different. I felt comfortable in this body that had just created another strand of our family lineage. The truth is, I had been doing the work quietly. I was starting to focus on me, how I felt, how I wanted to feel, how I saw myself, and who I wanted to be. I started to praise my body for what it has allowed me to do, to try, and to get through. I wish there was some magic workout or affirmation I could share, but it was tiny steps over a long time.

I was changing the thoughts in my head that had me playing small, questioning my worth, doubting and judging myself. I made a decision after becoming a mom that I wanted to raise strong, confident daughters, and in order to do that, I needed to be that. I needed them to see what it looked like. I wanted to be the example, not just the mom who told them to go after their dreams while denying my own, not the mom who told them how intelligent and capable they are while looking down on myself. I needed to live those values. I started acting on the things I wanted in life. I started building this muscle of confidence and consistency step by step. I started to recognize all the qualities I admired in myself, and I started to question my own thoughts, beliefs, and actions.

However, thoughts continued to tell me that exhaustion was normal in my effort to appear like a good wife, good mother, good person, but at the expense of feeling like a shell. I was going through the motions, but I was numb and burned out. I was showing up, but not in the way I wanted.

I was starting to pay attention to where and when I felt drained and frustrated. This confidence didn't just come from looking at myself in the mirror, which I did, or saying nice things to myself, which I also did. It didn't come from my husband treating me differently, because he has always showered me with affection and admired my curves. It came from doing—from doing the things I said I would do, the things that scared me a little. I started to keep my word to myself and trust that word again. I started with curiosity, with questions like: "What if I could?" "What or who could support me?" "How can this be easier?" "Why not me?" Slowly but surely, all of me just felt safe.

When the world changed in 2020, I was home full time like everyone else, and my work at a high-end hotel had closed temporarily. In May 2020, we found out I was pregnant, and I took my full year of maternity leave after giving birth. But I always saw myself working outside of my home, pursuing passions and connecting with interesting people daily (although I do consider myself an introvert, as I need to recharge by myself). I've been a massage therapist since 2006, became a trainer shortly after that, and while on my second maternity leave, I studied to become a health coach because I saw a need to help my clients outside of the four walls of a treatment room. Therefore, I chose an online course, studied every night when the kids were asleep, researched, took practice clients through a ninety-day transformation, and aced my exams. I came to health coaching because it combined all the things I loved about health and wellness with individualization, connection, and real-life strategies to help clients with things like burnout, chronic stress, blood sugar, and blood pressure, as well as building confidence, setting boundaries, and finding joy. I love using my mind and my body to help rid someone of physical pain and entertaining new ideas, connecting with their needs, their story, and their life experiences. Using my expertise, I build trust, exchange energy, and influence their physiology—how they breathe, sleep, move, and feel. There is something so magical about someone coming to you feeling stressed, stuck, and uncomfortable, then leaving with a clear plan and feeling inspired, supported, and pain-free.

My change from working at the hotel to being home full time caused me to be thankful that we had the finances to support us, but I also felt resentful—resentful toward my husband who was busier than ever in construction and working outside of the home, resentful because I was being a teacher, maid, caregiver, constant snack machine, cook, chauffeur, and mediator to my two older daughters, all while caring for a newborn. I was sleep deprived and perpetually needed by everyone all the time, while also trying to navigate building a business. Deep down inside I kept telling myself that I should love being home full time, but I felt guilt for wanting something different. No matter how hard I tried to be at peace with my life, I knew I still wanted to find a way to have space and time for myself and to have goals for my mission that had nothing to do with anyone else.

I had a choice. I could continue to wallow in overwhelm, or I could change my perspective, my expectations, and my approach. What if I just let go of the unrealistic ideals? What if I stopped expecting my life and my body to look like anything other than my own? I started to let go of what I thought I was supposed to be doing. I learned to be more present through ten-minute daily meditations and leaning into gratitude and the awareness that time is our greatest gift. I learned to question not just what I was feeling, but why. I explored whether I could change that feeling through listening to different coaches and applying the things I already knew. Moment by moment, day by day, even with the ups and downs of parenthood, marriage, and life, I got happier. I celebrated tiny wins. I felt more in control of my moods, my cravings, and my day. I didn't need anyone's approval, and I grew more aligned in my purpose.

Choosing not to go back to my comfortable job at the hotel was another step in growth. I wanted my own schedule and my own coaching program, and I longed to serve my community in a different way. My job didn't suit my needs or the needs of my family anymore. When they invited me back after my third maternity leave, I was so hesitant to make the final decision. Not returning would remove our financial safety net. I would be flying on my own, which would mean I was choosing my family, my business, and myself over the title, over the benefits, over the security, and over the familiarity of the job. It would also close a chapter that was instrumental in leading me to where I am today. The people I met there helped change my life, and I am grateful for that season, but I also know that seasons change and saying no to what didn't serve me anymore (ten hours a day away from home, the rigid schedule, the evenings and weekends away from my family) was an exercise of clarity and strength.

One of my biggest decisions recently was to go back into the clinic setting as an RMT. I felt like something was missing; something I enjoyed was gone. Yes, I had my regular private clients, but I wanted to work with a team again, to collaborate, and to get to know each client on a personal level. I struggled with the feeling because I felt that if I went back to massage therapy even part time, I would be turning my back on coaching, or worse, admitting that I'm not good enough to be a coach full time. But the truth is, being in that treatment room lights me up. Collaborating with chiropractors and physiotherapists, and getting to communicate with so many different people, helps me become a better, more compassionate therapist and coach. I have felt a shift in my presence, my energy, and my drive that has positively impacted my entire family. I am happier, and I get to do work I'm passionate about inside and outside of home. I get to show my family and my daughters what it looks like to build a life of service and success. I spent months making this decision, but ultimately, it has made me an abundantly better version of myself.

As a health professional, I feel it is part of my duty to practice what I preach, to walk my talk, and to show up in the best way possible. Going through the physical and emotional changes of motherhood and three pregnancies, existing in one body that has had multiple sizes and shapes, I pride myself in knowing what needs to be done to maintain a healthy mind and body. Knowing is not the same as doing—knowledge is helpful, but action is where the real change happens. Trial and error followed by lessons and growth. But learning to listen to my body has always been a work in progress. It has made me look at health, energy, and the interconnectedness of our systems in a new way that has benefited my clients. It has opened a road to re-educating myself in my body and relearning what I thought I knew. I've reconciled that as long as I am in this body, I'll have to relearn what serves me and what doesn't. This body has protected me, brought me through pain, and created life, and it allows me to interact with the world in meaningful ways. My physical, emotional, and spiritual bodies have been my light and dark. They have wisdom that I am learning to trust. Our body is our one true home, and this journey of becoming is what makes our stories unique.

I believe everything happens for a reason, even if I can't understand the meaning now. This journey was meant to change me, to teach me, to lead me to you, to affect me, to push me into another uncomfortable growth phase. It's not supposed to be easy; it's supposed to test me so I can blossom into my next evolution and be a safe space for women who are feeling how I have felt.

Now, if I close my eyes, I can feel the sun on my eyelids. I can see, hear, and smell that beach in Panama and feel that moment when I felt grounded, open, and vulnerable. Not everyone gets that chance, that moment to feel so deeply connected to self and earth, to purpose and meaning. That moment was a catalyst to bigger dreams, bigger possibilities, and a new way of seeing myself. It felt like that feeling was where I should live: in the energy of enough, the energy of possibility. When there is an opportunity that excites and scares you, that stretches and supports the future you envision, take it, soak it up, and take the lessons it serves.

This is my declaration of my possibility, of my meaning. Of my worthiness, strength, and grace. I hope you, too, can declare your possibility, your meaning. Be proud of your scars and your resilience, of your broken and your beautiful. You are enough because you are, because you were meant to be here. Whether I'm sitting on the floor with my kids, confidently coaching clients, helping relieve chronic pain, or sitting in some discomfort, I always have been and always will be enough, and so are you.

Chapter ELEVEN

When I Remembered Who I Was, the Game Changed

Lindsay Grace

There is such a shift in the world—we are opening up to our true power.

@thelindsaygrace

Lindsay Grace

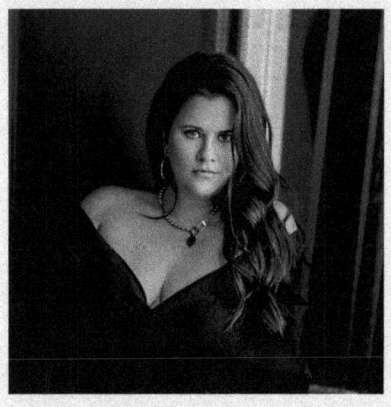

Lindsay Grace has mastered boldly living a life beyond her wildest dreams. She has the courage to follow her dreams, and she makes decisions that light her up. Lindsay helps others throw out the rule book, reclaim their power and worth, and remember who they truly are. She is gifted at reawakening the spirit inside others and reminding them of the path back to their own hearts and purpose. She believes that life doesn't have to be perfect, that it can be fun and messy, and she radiates the kind of energy that rips through BS narratives. Lindsay lovingly, yet with frightening honesty, shakes shit up. She has strength to move mountains, and she helps guide others to remember that they have it too.

INSTAGRAM @thelindsaygrace

To my brilliant kids, Kalman and Ella. You are my reason to heal and become the best version of me. I want you to see what is possible and how your life really can be everything you dream of.

When I Remembered Who I Was, the Game Changed

Have you ever felt like the universe was trying to send you a message? And maybe you weren't listening, so it kept getting louder and louder until one day it literally smacks you upside the head?

Well, that was me!

Ten years ago I thought I had it all figured out. I thought I had found my path and my people, my inner circle. I had a thriving business that I loved. I was being recognized as a successful mompreneur through the media, both for my business and myself. I was married and had two amazing kids. We had just moved back to my favorite area. I felt grounded and like I was home. Like for once, everything was going right.

This was beyond important to me, as we had just gone through many years of struggle. Everything you could imagine happening—family crumbling, job loss, financial struggle, our brand-new dream home becoming a disaster, six months of major health issues—happened, and little did I know that it was really only the beginning.

I had no clue at that time that all those random events occurring to us weren't so random.

It wasn't until the day that I was literally smacked in the head that

I started to question everything. I was in the prime of my life at the company's biggest social media conference, standing and chatting with a group of incredible businesswomen who I called my friends, when I was suddenly hit in the back of the head. I had no idea what had happened, and everyone started asking me if I was okay. I was so embarrassed and conditioned to not make a big deal of things that I automatically said yes.

Within a few minutes, however, I knew I wasn't okay, and that was the beginning of the end—a long drawn-out end. But that "end" was really only just the catalyst to major life changes and a ten-year journey in healing.

To the outside world, I had an incredible life. Very few people knew what was really going on behind closed doors, and that no matter what I achieved in my life, I still didn't feel right. I didn't know then what I know now. I lived a very holistic lifestyle: I focused on self-care, regularly worked with a healer, and had watched and read *The Secret*. I should've known all the things. What I didn't see then was that the most important lesson I would ever experience would put me onto the correct path: everything bad was happening so that I would wake up to my true purpose. But instead, I just dug my feet in even harder to try to make this world around me stop crumbling.

I began to think that maybe I just wasn't meant to have the kind of life that I aspired; that what other people had wasn't meant for me. After all the bad we had already experienced, then this: suffering a life-changing brain injury and closing the business I had lovingly built alongside raising my two babies. I had no idea what was left for me. Things got dark, I had no purpose, and I was so unhappy in my life. If it weren't for my kids, I don't know what the outcome would've been.

They were my reason to get up each morning and keep going. They were my world.

We've all heard the saying, "Everything happens for a reason," and it's true! Through those darkest times, all I knew was that there was a much bigger reason for it all, and while I didn't know what that reason was then, I would one day.

That smack in the head changed me. My brain shifted into a new way of living, thinking, and being. It activated my intuition to a level I didn't think was possible for me. But don't get me wrong; it wasn't an overnight switch. There were so many years of coincidences happening, but I still didn't tune in. I was living in the world tuned out from my inner self. I was living for everyone else, but not for me. And that was the reason I was so unhappy; it wasn't because of the brain injury.

This is what it means to be out of alignment.

But the truth is, the more my world crumbled, the more I dug in my feet to try to fix it. I did it all, but it didn't matter. I needed that to happen so that one day I finally woke up and realized that I didn't want to live like that anymore. That the life I wanted wasn't within the one I was living.

I was so scared, but I knew I had to finally end my marriage. I had spent twenty-six years with him, since age sixteen, and I didn't know a life beyond us. I had never been alone. I went from living at home to living with him. But the biggest wake-up call was that at age forty-two, I had no idea who I was. We hear people say that all the time, but for me, it was so true.

I will always remember how it felt that first weekend after my husband left. It was early and my kids were still sleeping so the house was quiet. I was folding laundry, and it just hit me: this is what it feels like to be free. I was excited! I was alone; it was just me. I could finally do anything and everything that I wanted without having to worry about anyone else. What would this open up for me?

In the midst of my divorce, my own spiritual healer said something that stuck with me: "This isn't going to be a new chapter in your book called life, this is going to be a completely new book." She has been one of my biggest supporters, both for me and my awakening. She is the connection to my own spirit guides and higher self, something so important as I worked to break through the past and the programming and started coming back home to me. I know now how important it is for healers to have their own healer.

So there I was, single and finally living life for me. I loved my alone time, but it was also hard. The world was suffering the effects of the pandemic and lockdowns, so I was forced to spend a lot of time alone, just me, and it was hard and lonely at times. But the lockdowns also allowed me to not distract myself with the busyness of life, something I was so good at doing. I had no choice but to face everything.

Don't let me fool you into thinking I was living this perfect utopian healing journey. At one point I was in weekly therapy, working with a life coach and my incredible spiritual healer. Being in lockdown catapulted my healing, my awakening, and my own self into my dark night of the soul. It also brought me what would be the thing that truly changed my life.

Remember how I said that the universe sends you messages? Well, it does! It will gently nudge us to things. Those seemingly random coincidences aren't so random. For weeks I had been seeing an ad on Facebook for a free webinar on how the Akashic Records and the laws of karma are the key to manifesting what we want. I had no idea what the Akashic Records were, but I had always felt that maybe I had bad karma. I used to sit and wonder who I'd pissed off, or who'd put a hex on me to keep having all the shitty stuff happening.

Then I thought that maybe I should watch the webinar. Why not? What did I have to lose? I've always been into self-help and learning how to be a better me. Maybe it was what I needed. So I signed up and waited for the following weekend when the webinar would be held. And during the hour-and-a-half presentation, I took notes and had constant aha moments. My entire life made sense! Sounds dramatic, but it was true.

In that time I learned that life doesn't just happen to us, how misunderstood karma is, and how it can be our best friend in manifestation. Yes, it is true that our actions have consequences, but it goes deeper than that. If we make a choice out of love, we get love. Out of fear, we get fear. Out of lack, we get lack. And all the choices I'd been making were based in fear or lack.

Oh my god, I'd created everything that had happened in my life, but it is so much more complex!

This webinar showed me that I needed to claim that. When we claim our mess, it is the only way out. The negativity in my life was because of something I created. Stuff doesn't just happen to us—we are not victims or powerless, even in a controlling relationship. I blamed my mess of a life and my unhappiness on everyone else, but it all really did come back to me. Harsh reality, but it was also the beginning of massive change in my life.

Consciousness and responsibility equal power.

We can't be both the powerful creators of some circumstances in our lives while other things just randomly happen. We are responsible for it all. Negative choices affect our ability to manifest. We also have to understand that they are only negative because they go against our divine self, and what might be negative for me might be incredibly positive for someone else, and vice versa. We often make choices for ourselves that we deem as positive because they are something we grew up with and learned from family or society, but they are actually negative. Standards we grew up with are not what we can use as the measure of a positive or negative choice for ourselves.

For me, staying in my marriage because I didn't want to be another divorce statistic (something I viewed as a big negative) was a big failure for me. But staying in an unhappy marriage would have been a negative choice. I wasn't able to live as my divine self in that marriage. I was so misaligned with my soul's purpose that I was always in a space of lack. And in the times I did live closer to it, there was always massive discord in the relationship.

The webinar dug deeper into the Akashic Records and the information that is contained in them. It spoke of a modality called Soul Realignment. This was all gibberish to me. I had never heard these terms before, and I was already living a holistic life where I was open to many different healing modalities. But I was looking for these modalities to heal me and believed that the spiritual wisdom sources from outside would tell me what to do. I didn't know then that spirit will never tell us what to do because free will is ours and asking won't get us a result.

In my original notes I had written "soul realignment training: look into this," and by the end of the webinar, I knew I had to sign up and learn. I needed to invest in this teaching. I had no plans to do anything more with this modality than that. When I looked at how much I had already spent on healing and therapy, I recognized that I had only been making tiny shifts. Yes, life was better, but in reality, I was so tired of feeling stuck and unhappy. I had made one of the biggest life changes, but I was still at a crossroads.

After all the work I had already done, I was still just functioning to fulfill everyone else's expectations of me. Fear, worries, and doubts were still in the forefront of my mind. People around me still had control and could push my buttons way too easily. I had trauma, lots of it. The fears were preventing me from moving forward into the next stage of my life.

Learning Soul Realignment was beyond life changing. In the first few weeks it showed me that there are two big keys keeping me from living the life I desired. First, it showed me how I wasn't living aligned to my highest path and purpose; I wasn't aligned to my Soul's divine blueprint. Remember back before my brain injury when I had that amazing business and life wasn't so bad? I was partially living my purpose then.

Second, it showed that people carry so much "baggage" from their lifetime, and even past lifetimes. This old baggage that no longer serves us is an energy block. We never really focus on the unpacking and actually getting rid of it, so it keeps us stuck in repeating cycles. It allowed me to see that past choices were still perpetuating, and it was like a massive blind spot in my life where I was still experiencing the consequences. It sifted through everything to help me understand how these patterns were still creating negative and very unwanted results.

I decided that I couldn't keep this learning for myself. There are so many others out there that need this, just like I did. Thus, I had to go all in and get my certification.

I struggled. It was hard learning. I wondered if my brain injury wouldn't allow me to really grasp it enough to do this work. I walked away from learning for months; I felt so defeated. I was resigned that once again, maybe my life was not meant to be what I really desired; maybe this was just as good as it would get for me, and that was okay.

It's a good thing I am stubborn and refuse to give up. I got on one of the support calls and told the teacher how I was struggling, and she helped me work through my block. This was part of my journey: seeing that I really could do anything I wanted, and that a brain injury wasn't going to hold me back.

When I finally did a Soul Realignment session on myself, I cried. Everything from the previous ten years made sense, and I couldn't believe that I might actually have the chance to change things. It's ironic to look back on it now because I really had no idea just how much things would change, not only for me, but for my clients. To receive my certification, I had to do this work on a group of practice clients, and their lives changed much faster than mine did.

See for me, I was still struggling to believe that my soul's purpose and gifts were actually mine. I am centered all around manifestation, building things, and power, yet I could not manifest and had no power. I know now that I could manifest; I was just manifesting all of the crap. It took me six months to realize that it really was me, and when things were okay in my life, it was because I was living part of that. I never had power that didn't exist in my life. I always felt that I had to make everyone else happy for me to be happy. I would give up my wants to keep peace. I gave up my power. That is a big no for me. My soul needs it, and it's something I will never give up again.

I remember driving down the highway to the car dealership to buy my new car when a thought struck me: what I was doing worked, and the key was just living my soul-aligned life! We really are the powerful creators of our lives. I'd manifested the new car in a month, all on my own, the car I dreamed of and didn't really think was possible for me. The brain injury, being on disability, and my divorce had almost financially destroyed me. How could I possibly buy a brand-new Audi SUV? And all on my own? I was starting to magnetize and pull everything I desired to me.

I started seeing my worth, something that when I look back, I really never had. This healing journey, and the clearing all my baggage, allowed me to go back in time to when I was sixteen and made the decisions I did for my life. Holding space for that teenage version allowed me to build the foundation of self-worth.

There is such a shift in the world—we are opening up to our true power. We understand more and more that we really are in complete control of our lives. Through this I have seen, and not only in myself but in all those around me, that we are taking control of our healing. We are trying so many different modalities and incorporating self-care and self-love into our everyday lives and routines. Look at how many people you know who are using natural products, crystals, and meditation. Collectively, there is a desire for deep knowing of who we are. We understand that there is so much more to this universe than we thought, than we grew up with. This movement is healing generations of trauma, for our ancestors, for ourselves, and for our kids.

Throughout the past three years I have healed more than I could've fathomed. I have gone deep into Soul Realignment and the wealth of knowledge available to us in the Akashic Records. In recognizing that we are energetic beings, and when we start with us, our entire external world changes. I have learned human design and how to embrace our shadows—they are a part of us and our magic. I have learned all about frequency and vibration and how we can utilize it to help support our healing, and by doing this, we are also assisting in the healing of the collective.

This new me, this life, is something I created. I want to help others see that they can too.

Chapter TWELVE

Clearing the Fog

Jessica Callery

Life can feel scary and dark, but I now know that the fog will lift and that the sun will shine again.

@jessica.heaven_ @jessicacallerycoaching

Jessica Callery

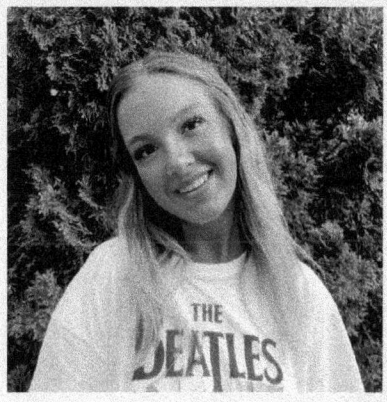

Jessica Callery is a mother of two and an intuitive mindset coach, author, creative, and mental health advocate. Her mission is to help others by being vulnerable about her own story. Jessica is driven by making people feel connected, and her next project will be writing her own book.

INSTAGRAM @jessica.heaven_ @jessicacallerycoaching

For all the lost souls out there, I promise there is a way home.

Clearing the Fog

I was basking in the sunlight, curled up in my favorite flannel blanket with a cup of orange pekoe. My thoughts were melancholy and in a pitiful demise. I was discouraged. Was I broken? What I would learn quickly is there is a hero and a villain in every story, and they are often the same person.

Grandma Helen always reminds me that the day I was born was foggy, and I grew up in a fog most days once I hit double digits. But when I was born, the world was so angelic, pure, and open with possibilities through my big brown eyes. It's kind of strange, isn't it? How we are born with no idea what's to come and no control over it either? Little Jessica had no idea the obstacles, grief, and loss she would endure.

My connection to Spirit was always waiting to beam out. As a little girl, I felt something outside myself I could not explain. I felt this outside source of magnetic energy that swirled around my body, just out of reach, but in my skin and bones. Because I didn't have a grip on how to tap into this outside energy that surrounded my aura, it manifested in my body as anxiety and feelings of depletion, like I did not know my own thoughts. I couldn't articulate what was happening inside my mind and body; I felt completely detached and like an alien from a different dimension.

I remember being at summer camp when I was around ten and having crippling anxiety with no explanation or reasoning. I just felt so many things. Heard so many things. It was like intrusive messaging I heard but did not know what it was or how to process it.

As I grew up, and specifically after losing my dad, I connected on a different level I never knew possible and was then able to understand my spiritual gifts more. I learned that there was a name to what I had been experiencing since I was a child: I was clairaudient. Becoming spiritually well again was my key to freedom. I missed the reality and the beauty of my gifts because I was diverted by the ugliness of my trauma. Being able to recognize that I could use these gifts for good and it was not just my grief coming up would be my ticket to freedom and clearing the fog.

My childhood years are a mix of experiences, some remembered, some forgotten, some possibly blocked because they are too painful. When I look back now, I truly feel there were anxieties and fears already in me that at the time I had no idea, perhaps, how to handle. Nobody spoke of anxiety, and mental health wasn't a topic one heard about. Many people, including myself, suffered in silence. I can't go back in time and fix it, but I can give myself grace to know I did not have the coping skills to deal with it. As the years went on and my anxiety increased, I reached for anything that would numb my pain: drugs, alcohol, sex . . . anything that would take me out of reality. My spirituality was in a fog: I was pushing down all of me because I could not handle myself. I can find forgiveness in myself for doing all I knew how to at the time. This revelation has helped me not only find support for myself but also turn it into a passion to support others.

Life sure is a funny thing when you think about it. What I once thought would break me has made me a better person. I have more insight into the world of addiction and mental health than I would never have known without my own unique experiences. As a child, you are given certain experiences through no choice of your own: where you live, who you live with, what you see or don't is not in your control. What is in your control is what you do with this information as an adult. I had to realize at some point to hold onto the good memories and experiences as a child while letting go of or, at a minimum, accepting the experiences I didn't enjoy or choose and decide to change that going forward. I could now choose to be who I wanted and have full power and control of what that would look like. How freeing is that? I had to decide it didn't matter what time had passed. I had the knowledge to make the change and take a different path, one out of the fog. And when I chose that path, it was the greatest joy and feeling. I was in charge of my own destiny!

Painful events shape us all. I eventually realized that I could transmute my most painful experiences into the very pillars of my strength. When I lost my dad at fourteen, I saw myself as broken, something that made me empathetic and cherish life. When my stepdad committed suicide, all I saw was confusion, anger, and sadness, all emotions that made me compassionate about mental health. When suffering through an abusive relationship, all I felt was worthless, a feeling that made me independent and stand up for domestic violence. Being sexually assaulted and feeling used made me respectful of bodies. Being addicted to cocaine and alcohol and feeling useless and pathetic made me understand addiction and discover who I was. My purpose. All these things made me a better, stronger, wiser, braver version of myself.

I used to let these things keep me down. My trauma is not my excuse to drink. It is one of the reasons why a sober lifestyle is a suitable choice for me. When I tend to my mind and find a peaceful solution, that is where the magic happens. Now I share my light with the world by helping those who have dealt with similar situations tap into their spirituality. Your darkness really is your light. Although time is ongoing, you can stop the clock. Look at all you have done and overcome when you turn the clock backward. You've climbed mountains. I was finally giving devotion to the things inside me that required nurturing. You can do it too. Anything is possible. I am not broken; I am imperfectly me. You are not broken; you are imperfectly you.

Thankfully, I no longer wallow in pity or try to escape reality. I sit in the mess. I will do whatever it takes to come out from the pain. Sometimes life is like walking through the thickest fog with no idea what's to come. Life can feel scary and dark, but I now know that the fog will lift and that the sun will shine again. This does not mean the pain goes away, but you can find the light and use your story for good. It is possible to go from darkness to lightness. There is light. So let there be light.

In 2022 I finally let that light blind me. This time I would relish it. I would taste it, smell it, see it for all it was. I was beginning my journey of becoming alcohol-free. Quite honestly, I had attempted sobriety more times than I could count; this time, however, something was equivocally different. My mind knew I could not drink and was uncomfortable with how my thought process was in terms of alcohol. I was surrounded by fog when I would drink. Nothing seemed clear anymore, and I would lose sight of my authentic self.

This was my road to freedom. The things I thought were darkness have turned into my light. When I open my heart and speak my truth, I am free. I am helping those who suffer in silence to open up. In surrendering to something that does not serve me, I suddenly was on different footing. My roots grasped a new soil, and my mind, body, and soul felt much more inwardly reorganized. It truly was a rebirth. The effect this metamorphosis had was electric. I had alchemized my pain, trauma, experiences, and anger. At last, it was safe to be me. The self-awareness I had come to know was before my eyes. My eyes welled up in this moment that I will never forget: a literal beam of light flashed before my eyes, and a distinctive, clear, peaceful voice said that to be honest with thine self means you are free. I had utterly and shamelessly confessed all my deepest, darkest secrets to myself. All that mattered is what I felt about them. I had been searching for something outside myself that was in me all along. I had far too many warnings I had failed to acknowledge wholeheartedly, but something struck a chord this time and I was set free. I was unapologetically myself inside every bone in my body.

This was not only a pathway of freedom for myself but also for my spiritual gifts—I was now clear of the fog. The fog that had followed me for so long was finally lifted. At last, I could honor myself and my role in the world around me. I was beaming wide open and set free. This clarity would come to shape the rest of my life.

I acknowledge that all my experiences thus far have made me who I am. Throughout the fog there was a light trying to shine. I am grateful that the sunlight within my soul has finally returned home. I release the anger that was holding me hostage and no longer feel such darkness seeping into my life. The disconnect between myself and the beam of light that shines within me is finally one. As each day passes, I feel stronger and stronger. This is my biggest gift right now. Being thankful for this chance to come into my own and share with others with no fear of judgment and being proud of who I am and where I am going. Although I have done many shameful things, I am not ashamed of who I am. I have ripped myself open and unmasked every limb, bone, and dirty secret that was alive inside me, and I have accepted it all. The good and the bad, my weaknesses and my strengths, and just truly being Jessica. I promise you it will never work trying to be someone you are not. Today, I am unapologetically and authentically me. This makes me feel lighter and lifts a heaviness I never even knew was the weight that held me down.

Chapter THIRTEEN

She Who Chased

Jenny Bitner

When we can begin to connect back to our source of power, miracles start to happen every day in every way.

@iamjennybitner

Jenny Bitner

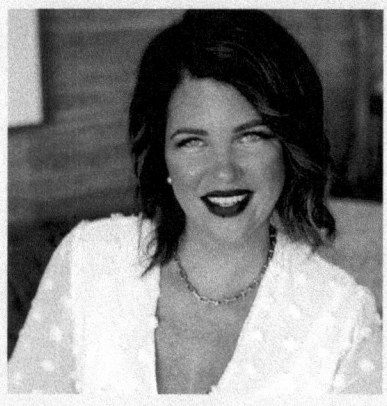

Jenny Bitner is a keynote speaker, director of fun, and ever-evolving student of the power of the Mind. After a decade as a top-performing corporate general manager who gave up her career due to executive burnout, Jenny had the idea that freedom would be found in entrepreneurship. Eight years and building three business models to six-figures later, she noticed her tendency to push herself into exhaustion and fatigue was a deeply ingrained habit, not a job requirement. She had her lightbulb moment when it struck her that work isn't just about making money, it's about having FUN while doing it! Now Jenny is consulting with visionary leaders and companies that desire to build team environments where Profit meets PLAY™. She believes the best-trained teams win and a learning experience on the frequency of fun brings the embodiment of freedom and success to everyone.

INSTAGRAM @iamjennybitner

To my loving and spirited diva, Paislee, and my fierce warrior, Everlee Joy: my two blue-eyed little minis who will know life is about memories over money and that the greatest success is finding your truth and inner wisdom.

She Who Chased

I proudly handed my dad my Grade 12 report card: 88 percent average.

He looked at me with slight disappointment and asked, "Where can you make up the twelve percent?"

I've always remembered this moment because of how deflated I felt when I realized that if I wasn't perfect, it was a reflection of my worth. When there was something I could've been better at, I would always feel that disappointment in myself. I don't blame my dad's role in this, though. In fact, it was because of his belief in his children's capabilities that we turned out to be powerhouses. I know his intention was to have us strive to be the best that we could be, and that intention imprinted a negative thought cycle that caused me to spend years aiming for perfection and being hard on myself when I fell short.

The vice president of the company I worked for came into my office the same year I was nominated for General Manager of the Year. She handed me my sales audit—a 98 percent. I looked at her in sheer disappointment. "Where could I have made up the two percent?" I asked.

Our whole lives, we are shaped. Specifically:

- Social heredity tells us how to act and behave and what is right and wrong.
- Teachers spend thirty+ hours a week with us for ten months a year, shaping our psyche.
- Parents, doing the best they can, pass on generational beliefs and coding.
- Media shapes our minds from a young age.
- Religion instills certain belief systems and keeps us following a specific path.

We spend a lifetime trying to appease those in authority positions, making them proud and seeking validation for being "good." Everyone is doing their best to raise us to be our best. We work with what we have, and to paraphrase Maya Angelou, when we know better, we do better (at least, that's what we hope).

I was always the one who did whatever possible to make my authority figures proud. I worked hard, I showed up, I put in the most effort, I did things according to direction. My desire to be seen in the highest regard left me yearning for the attention and pride of those from whom I sought the most assurance.

I was the girl who chased the awards, accolades, rewards, recognition, and validation. The only way I ever felt that I had made it was by being recognized by other people. In friendships, I chased love, acceptance, and the validation that I was good enough. In school, then business, the only way I knew whether I had manifested success for myself was when somebody else gave me the title for it.

Although this moving target kept me fairly well focused on my goals, it also made me incredibly vulnerable to attack-and-doubt thoughts,

thoughts that stem from our lower mind. They create the fear that steadily creeps in and wreaks havoc on our ability to perceive ourselves as perfectly whole.

Following my graduation from university, I got a job in sales for the largest chain of fitness clubs in Canada in order to bridge the time before my acceptance into teacher's college in Australia. Within a few months I became the top consultant in the entire country.

My ego kicked in and I began the chase.

I worked fourteen-hour days, drinking copious amounts of coffee and running myself into the ground, just to keep that top rank. I was competing for the dream vacations, the incentives, and the prized nomination companywide at the end of the year.

Six months into the job, I was diagnosed with a severe anxiety and panic disorder. I started off having a few panic attacks here and there, which then manifested into my having multiple attacks a day with a side dish of chronic anxiety. I lived with this condition for more than a decade. It took root in every area of my life and began to set up permanent camp in my mind. I had zero clue what to do about it, and the "help" out there was barely enough to even touch this beast.

Throughout my twenties and thirties, I lived a life of duality: on one side I was running a multimillion-dollar fitness club and winning awards for my achievements, but on the flip side, I was hiding in my office with the door locked, trying to recover from multiple panic attacks a day.

I knew this was not a healthy way to live, but at the time, no one at work seemed to be talking about it. So, I decided to speak up, and as it turned out, I was not the only one feeling that way.

In fact, almost every other manager felt the intense pressure, the endless strive for reaching goals, and the aching disappointment when they weren't achieved. They, too, felt anxious if another month of low sales would pass and wondered whether they would lose their job as a result. I don't believe it was the company imposing this atmosphere; rather, it was a societal norm at that time: hustle and grind.

Listen, I'm not opposed to having a stellar work ethic; in fact, I am the poster girl for perseverance and dedication to my craft. But what if it could feel good in the process?

When I began to lose joy in my days, I knew something had to change. Eventually, I realized that the reason my body and mind were in disharmony was because all my worth was externally driven. I had given all my power to the attack-and-doubt thoughts instead of harnessing the inner teacher that had been silenced for all those years.

I have far too many memories of when my desire to be accepted and chosen outweighed my alignment: I chose money over family; I chose acceptance over being with those I truly felt inspired being around; I chose a place where there was more opportunity for recognition over doing something that I loved.

No matter how much success I had, there was always a void. Nothing ever felt good enough, the chase never seemed to end, and there was no feeling of satisfaction. I just dumped all my hard work into a bottomless bucket, and I never seemed to fill my cup.

I had not learned by that point that my mind is my most precious resource, and if used correctly, it could take me to heaven on earth. And once I tapped into the power and miracles that opened up when my mind became the entire focus for how I navigated my life, everything changed.

A few years ago, I began to learn about two different thought systems.

When I dove into the self-education behind our purpose on this planet, how to leverage the mind and the body, and what is what and who is who, all the lightbulbs started turning on. I looked around and realized that we are all in this dream. We all have the same power, but so many of us are sleeping. When we can begin to connect back to our source of power, miracles start to happen every day in every way.

Let's just touch the surface here. As I mentioned, there are two thought systems. Now, these thought systems can only be operated one at a time, so it's imperative that we understand each of them so we can make the choice that best suits our life and know how that decision will affect the perception and the lens through which we see the world. Allow me to take you through this journey of opening your mind to the decision that we have been given as human beings.

When I was in the deepest valley of my panic and anxiety disorder, I was operating out of a thought system that was driven by my ego. It was the lower part of my mind. It was the part of my mind that operated from fear and guilt and shame. I lived my life from a place where I was always looking out for ways to avoid situations that would cause my body to experience major distress.

I lived my life ensuring that everything I did made others proud. If I was about to do something that had the potential to impact my reputation in a negative way, I removed myself within seconds, as I would have thoughts that filled my lower mind: *What will others think? How will other people judge me? What is this going to look like from the outside? How is this going to impact the potential of me moving up in my job? How will this decision impact the way that another person might talk about me?* Everything that I did was measured up against: *How will it make me look?* rather than *How does this make me feel?*

I lived my life through a lens where the world was harmful and scary and every move I made could have a negative impact on me. My nervous system was operating in a chaotic space, and I rarely felt calm and grounded. Once I started learning about the mind and the power of our thoughts, however, a door opened and provided me with the opportunity to change the lens.

The new lens is one that is perceived through the higher mind. So, if the lower mind is the ego, the higher mind is the one connected to our source.

Let me explain the mind this way:

Think of the sun. Typically, when we draw the sun, we draw a big yellow circle with lots of rays coming off it. I want you to imagine that at the end of each one of those rays coming from that fiery ball of energy is a little human body.

The mind is the sun: the main mind, the source, the original place from which all eight billion rays (people) come. Thus, a fragment of that mind is in every single human. The body is the vessel, the tool that encapsulates this mind so that people can walk around the earth, see each other, have a human experience, and interact. And yet, we all share the exact same mind.

Being on earth as humans gives us the opportunity to experience a duality that we couldn't experience if we were just a mind alone in all its perfect purity. As humans, we have the opportunity to experience a life where we have the autonomy to choose from one of two thought systems. We all have the higher mind and the access to the higher mind, which is what connects us all to source. The higher mind is in every single human being, and it is the ray of sun that connects us. It is the path to all miracles.

The sun is nothing but pure, potent, powerful, loving energy. But because we're human, we also have access to a lower mind, which is the duality. The lower mind is the ego and the part of our mind that can access fear, guilt, and shame. It is important to note that it is an illusion; it's not part of the real love of the original source, the sun. Having this lower part of our mind, this ego, this access to the duality of feeling emotions that can bring about experiences, separates us from the higher mind. We cannot possibly operate out of both minds simultaneously. So, with every single decision we make every single day, we are choosing which part of the mind to use.

You can even ask yourself: *In this moment, am I using my higher mind to bring me closer to my source, closer to love, closer to joy, closer to peace of mind? Or am I perceiving the world out of the lens of the lower mind of the ego, where I'm feeling fear, where I'm feeling guilt, where I'm feeling shame?* The lower mind has been corrupted in this world.

When we learn how the power of the mind can impact every single moment of our life, we can finally unlock the codes to every mind miracle that can be experienced every day.

One of the ways I have shifted away from a life where I was chasing the money, chasing the awards, chasing the recognition, and chasing the validation is to begin looking at what I ultimately desired.

Let's take money as an example. Most people desire two things: money and peace of mind—money because it removes scarcity or lack of security, allowing us to feel safe and secure in taking care of ourselves and our family; it allows us to have access to the things that we desire. But money means nothing if we don't have peace of mind, a mind that is not chaotic, loud, or flustered with intrusive thoughts. Peace of mind is the most important value for bringing people into the highest frequency possible.

When I began my journey back to my inner teacher, I asked myself how I would be able to move from just *desiring money* (because others are making big money and I want to too) and buying luxurious items to creating an abundance of peace-of-mind wealth.

Well, being a spiritual ministry student of A Course in Miracles has changed everything for me.

I have learned that "things," well, all materialism, is just an illusion. The actual purpose of this human experience is to raise ourselves up the emotional and energetic frequency scale from a place of fear, shame, and guilt to a place where we can achieve joy, peace of mind, and enlightenment. Enlightenment is the highest energetic frequency on this planet, and it's where we can connect to our source effortlessly. Can you imagine having the purest, most direct contact with our "sun"?

When I was operating in the lower mind, when I had addictions to the materialism, to the chase, my frequency was vibrating so low that I was an energetic match for experiences that would keep me in a perpetual spinning state of anxiety, panic, uncertainty—states that made me feel unsafe.

As I learned how to shift to my higher mind and began to make a channel directly to source, I was able to lift up the sensations in my body that didn't feel good. I lifted thoughts that weren't pure and asked my source to purify them. I also asked the source to move the sensations out of my physical body and to lift them up where they would be light as a feather.

This practice took years to embody because I was only understanding piece by piece the truth of what is available to us. In the past twelve months alone, I have unraveled so much of my ego that I have experienced what can be called an ego death. I have begged and prayed to God to remove the attachment I have had on money and materialism and to replace it with the desire—the obsessional desire—for memories, for moments with my family and experiences that bring me more joy.

And through this process, I have removed the people, the places, and the experiences that no longer serve my higher mind. I've begun to unravel from an unhealthy masculine energy and am allowing my sacred feminine energy to come through. But I'm not going lie: I've fought this process, as it's been challenging. It's led me to breakdowns, tantrums, crying fits, and even feelings of depression at times. But every single moment along the way, I've known with unshakable certainty that this is the ego's death. This is the opening of my channel straight to source. This is the purification of me. And in realizing that this is actually the purpose of the human experience, and in embracing it, I am welcoming in moments that allow me to put these lessons to the test. I've embraced this challenge with an open heart and an open crown, so that I can allow that purification to sink into my physical body.

Now, don't get me wrong: I still have my days. I am human like you and every other person on this planet (well, that's debatable, but we'll save that story for another book!). There are still things I do to accommodate the thought patterns that are linked back to my old anxiety. There are things I do to keep myself comfortable when traveling so I do not expose myself to old patterns that have residual coding in my cells.

I, like you, am a beautiful work in progress. I will continue to place myself in experiences that allow me to practice my surrender and have faith that when I choose my higher mind, I am safe and taken care of.

No one is perfect. If we were, we wouldn't be in a body experiencing this life on earth. We were given the chance to come here to feel the separation and duality of emotions. We have been given the chance to learn how to raise our frequency and manifest all we desire. We have it in us to connect to source, to ask for what we want, and to be held in pure love. We hold the power to forgive, to attune to our inner teacher, to practice deep faith and trust, and . . . to experience miracles.

I no longer need validation, or a sense of security, from anything or anyone outside of myself. This was a journey back home that took grit. And it also took a sense of commitment to the undoing. It took commitment to unraveling and to holding it all along the way, and it took welcoming in love. As I walk my truest path to the highest frequency available to me in this human experience, it is my hope that others will begin to see the light and make their journey back home as well.

I have gone from chasing money, validation, recognition, and achievements to chasing the light back to the sun.

Chapter FOURTEEN

Uniting Two Worlds

Nicole Campagna

For me to do a job well, I have to be myself.

*@howwomen_*

Nicole Campagna

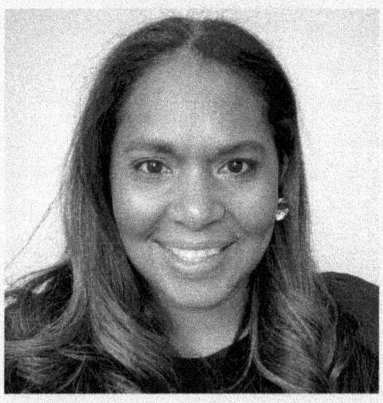

Nicole Campagna is committed to and passionate toward all things people related in the workplace. A mom of three boys and a leader within human resources, Nicole brings her whole self wherever she can in all her experiences and relationships. She is energized when connecting and collaborating with others who have a strong purpose and shared values. Driven by a constant curiosity to learn and unlearn, Nicole is committed to a journey of developing herself and others whenever and wherever she can. Nicole is also the founder of How Women, a supportive community and network of women to support their leadership journey of professional and personal growth.

INSTAGRAM @howwomen_

To my village, to every human who has provided me with both the reason and the opportunity to get to this place, to find my way. And for everyone else still on their journey, keep going; you're almost there.

Uniting Two Worlds

It is a story we hear far too often: women and mothers resorting to making a choice—a choice between their career and the life they envisioned as a mother. Each and every story is unique. A story where hopefully the individual gets to a place where she finds balance in achieving her intended goals.

In some of these situations it may mean leaving a job in a workplace, taking strengths and interests and translating them to create the business of her dreams, working for herself, and creating a life on her terms. Not necessarily working more or fewer hours but finding the flexibility to give her more influence and control over her schedule and decisions.

And there are also other stories of courage, of women who chose to leave the life of working for someone else in a traditional workplace environment and dedicate their available time and hours to their families and as a mother. You will notice that I emphasize the decision of time allocation versus a decision on whether to abandon a career and choose a life as a full-time mother. Because that is not what is happening. I avoid the term "stay-at-home" when referring to a woman who has chosen to dedicate her time solely to her family. Because we all know that whether or not there is a salary attached to this work, women who have chosen to dedicate their time to being a mother are still working women. These decisions are usually based on an allocation of time. How a woman chooses to balance the limited hours in a day. In all these stories, we are not relinquishing our roles as mothers, nor are we abandoning our ambition to achieve occupational success, but our journey to get to our perfect balance and find our way home is what makes us different. A life built on priorities determined by us. These are great stories, inspiring ones.

In the words to follow I share with you my own story, another pathway, one I did not know existed and where a simple statement and the unfolding of a global pandemic changed where my story could have ended up and how I came home earlier than planned.

Let's turn back time to August 2017, to an experience that many women go through: the infamous return to work from maternity leave. There's anxiety over trying to figure out how I am going to make this work. Functioning off fewer than the recommended eight hours of sleep, I began planning: waking up early enough to make healthy lunches for the entire family, getting two kids off to school and a toddler to daycare, getting myself dressed (at a standard that had now changed from leggings, hoodies, and a high bun), thinking about dinner plans, then mentally preparing for a day at work. *Do I have enough gas in the car? Can I leave an extra ten minutes to do that and still make my first meeting? Is preparation required for my morning meeting? Do I have time to write a few emails while making breakfast?* (Before I continue, I must acknowledge that I, and my family, are incredibly blessed to have a very strong support system. It truly does take a village. I am definitely not doing this all by myself; even just thinking about it makes me realize that it is physically impossible to do any of this alone.) However, back in 2017, the mental load of *feeling* responsible for the coordination of everything, ensuring all the details were taken care of, still rested with me. The feeling that I needed to be present in many places and roles simultaneously.

This is where I found myself showing up as two different versions of me. In addition to all the logistic details required to maintain these two versions of myself, there was also the internal conflict. I was showing up at work every morning ready to be someone else. It was still me, but just not the same me. I have been fortunate to have always worked in an environment that respected a healthy work–life balance (for the most part), where life milestones were celebrated, partners and families were included in events, and colleagues knew your kids' names and ages and celebrated your life outside of work. Additionally, time off to care for or be with your family was respected. So, while there was no direct or overt judgment, it was perhaps still implied.

Walking out the office doors, saying goodbye to colleagues, wishing them a good evening, and joking about "starting your next job" was common, and a reality. The commute home was an opportunity to catch up on thoughts, to have a conversation with a friend or two, or to listen to a podcast or an audiobook, all while mentally preparing for the evening duties and before walking through the door at home and turning back into the other role, as a mother, while also overcompensating for all that I had missed during the day as that mother.

So, let's come back to that "different" me. Who is she? She's like many of us: a woman working to represent herself physically and characteristically as anyone other than a mother. At times, based on pressure from others, I dressed in ways outside my comfort zone and preferred style and made weekly appointments for a blowout to avoid the distraction of my frizzy, curly hair, all because it was what was expected of me. In the workplace, there is an unspoken rule that while being a mother can be part of our identity, it should not be who we are completely, nor should it be a barrier to our successes in the corporate environment. Who imposes this judgment or expectation on us? There is an assumption that it is always men that we are "hiding" from, but it is more complex than that. It is also from our female peers: those who have come before us, as well as those who will follow in the paths we pave behind us. The future us, the women who feel like they have already made it work and figured it out, while incredibly supportive, impose the expectation that if they could do it, so should we. And other women to whom we are their future. We work to inspire them, to be the role models who show them the possibility of being able to do it all. In most cases, women are our greatest allies, but they can also be our rivals.

And this is why I thought my only option was to continue to chase my entrepreneurial dream. I always knew I had the ambition, drive, and creativity to work for myself and build a business. Over the years, even before I started a family, I was always coming up with ideas or services to address a perceived gap or need. But for some reason, I couldn't cross the line and turn it from a side hustle to a full-time business. Even though I longed for the flexibility to be there for my family, I could not officially relinquish the connection to the corporate environment, the security, the structure, and the community of people.

When did the lightbulb flick on? Or actually, when did the lighthouse turn on? I was sitting in the corner boardroom with the executive team, the much sought-after spot by many women in my type of position and level within the organization. I had earned the desired "seat at the table." We aspire to be at the table, but what does the table represent? Who are we when we pull out the chair and take a seat? Where we sit, when we speak, what we say? These are all thoughts that run through our mind. Who should I be and represent in this chair to ensure I am accepted and respected?

At this particular table, in this boardroom encased by glass walls, the executive team gathered. I had been asked to prepare a process for the management team based on the direction they provided. We were in a highly sensitive situation and the articulation of each step of the process needed to be well thought out considering the implications of a misstep and the importance of the communication channels for certain situations. One of my identified strengths among this group was my creativity and use of progressive tools and applications to represent data. I was asked to prepare the initial draft and the accompanying communication.

It was my moment to process the information, create an impressive presentation, and communicate it to the stakeholders. I thought through the exercise from every perspective. In addition to creating the process map, I included specific directives for the managers based on my knowledge of the questions they would receive from their employees, as well as the questions they would have for the executive team and HR. Being in HR gives you a perspective and vantage point to the challenges, questions, and situations that managers face. My focus was to ensure they were equipped with the tools and information to navigate a complex situation. And most importantly, the managers needed to understand their roles in the process. The moment came. I walked into the room and connected my laptop to the screen. Before I presented, I reviewed the objective of the exercise and then launched into it. So proud, so confident, so sure. I relied on my judgment to execute the task. Managing the process and ensuring the expectations of the management team were clearly articulated. The executives listened, reviewed the information, paused, looked at me, reflected on what they were seeing, then with one statement, everything changed:

"This looks good, but it is too much information. You should remove some of these steps. You're mothering them."

Huh? Mothering them? What does that even mean? I wanted to shrink down to half my size and curl up under the table. Everything I had avoided representing in the corporate world was being thrown at me, and in a negative way. I have no doubt that the constructive feedback they provided was likely quite valid. I had overmanaged the situation. But it was the descriptive term used to articulate this feedback. My work was perceived to be inefficient and ineffective. I was filled with emotions. I was confused, embarrassed, and ashamed. My contributions were compared to a position where I make mac and cheese five times a week, change diapers, and pick socks off the floor. Oh wait, it was also the position where I received at least twenty hugs a day without request, the position where I am recognized for the love and compassion I bring to the situation and am appreciated for being me.

I relive this moment over quite a bit, reflecting on its implication on my story and how it changed my entire mindset on who I was supposed to be in both these worlds. Reflecting back, I should have been proud that someone described me and my skills as a mother. It is a role and position that I am incredibly proud of, and it is a role that I have experienced so much growth in and reward for throughout the past fourteen years. It is a role that I am immersed in 24/7. So why would I assume that I would think differently between the hours of 9 and 5 p.m. every day? When it came time to tap into an area of myself or one of my greatest strengths, doesn't it make most sense that I connected to a collection of skills that I felt most comfortable in? My parenting skills, where I was idolized, respected, and appreciated—a role where my team (my three sons) imposed no judgment of my skills.

But when I heard those words, my initial feeling was shame. As if my cover had been blown. And in that moment, why was the descriptor utilized in a negative tone? Why do we shy away from expressing ourselves authentically in these functions and tap into the strengths from no matter where they arise? Who I am as a contributor in the workplace has changed immensely during the years I have grown and evolved as a parent. I have strengthened and developed skills in time management, in communicating with impact and empathy to emotional needs, in delivering results and achieving objectives, in problem solving, and in so much more.

As parents, we spend time, whether consciously or not, reflecting on our values and principles. We work with our partners, communities, and support systems to ensure our children are being raised with specific values. Doesn't it make sense that they also be applied in the workplace? Why had I been working so hard to separate my two worlds for so long? Why wouldn't I bring my one true self to work?

Being in HR provided me with the opportunity to spend my days surrounded by other leaders and managers who were also parents, many of whom I knew in both their worlds. I observed managers who had a leadership style that was so different from who they were at home and as parents. I saw them struggle to find their place in their professional life. Now that I know more about these behaviors and realize the reasons, I can see they were not bringing their full, authentic selves to the workplace.

I am passionate and dedicated to all things people related in the workplace. I am constantly fascinated by human interactions in the work environment and am drawn to any activity that provides me with the opportunity to contribute in creating healthy workplaces and working relationships, which I guess is a good match and likely a prerequisite for being in HR and a leader within an organization. Being inside the organization, understanding needs, knowing the workplace culture, and getting to know the people is where I am supposed to be. I support managers and leaders wherever I can by being there for their teams and employees. But what I have learned is that for me to do that job well, I have to be myself, not the version of me that was expected of me. I realized that the reason I felt burned out or longed for a desire to find something else (as an entrepreneur) that was better suited for me was a reflection of who I was showing up as at work.

So where does the pandemic fit into all this? In a time when there's so much conversation about the importance of boundaries and the impact of the blurred lines between our work and home lives, I realized that the pandemic also forced us to be more of the same person, the true authentic version of ourselves, in both worlds. We had no choice. There was no time to turn off and then back on again. We were in survival mode: just do, just be. Zoom call after Zoom call, our work colleagues were inside our homes every day. Kids walking in and out of meetings, doorbells ringing when the Amazon packages arrived, pets walking across keyboards, hoodies worn as the office dress code. And, of course, we had the simultaneous dual role as teachers for online school. But we must remember that the reverse also had and continues to have implications. Really good ones. Our children saw a new side of us as parents. This new generation of children is being exposed to working parents who show them what they do when not being their mom or dad.

I was chasing the entrepreneur dream because I assumed that life would provide me with the opportunity to be myself. That by working for myself, I could be "me." I would have an environment where I wouldn't need to fit into a mold or assimilate into a situation or environment that was not a match for me. But between the pandemic and getting to a place where finding an environment that really allows me to be me, I realized where I belonged and where I knew I could and would thrive. Hiding the most important and authentic elements of myself, which are a collection of my experiences and behaviors (including being an awesome mom), is not an option.

For the first time in a long time, I finally feel like I am finding my place. My comfort zone. My identity as a parent and as a leader. While they are the best roles I have ever held, they are also the toughest, most important ones, and my having them is a privilege I do not take for granted. And when I say I have come home and found my comfort zone, it most certainly does not mean that I have figured it all out. But what I know more today than I have ever known is the role I want to play in the lives of my children and with my teams and within the organizations I support. I know the type of parent and leader I want to be. And there is not much difference in these roles. The "Nicole" you meet in the workplace (HR leader, manager, colleague) and the "Nicole" you'll find outside of work (wife, mom, daughter, friend, sister) are one and the same. My actual duties may be different, but who I show up as in each of those activities is the same. I am driven by values and creating experiences that I am proud to reflect on. I am no longer trying to be someone else or assimilate into an environment predetermined by someone else. And in using my learnings from these experiences, I am now more than ever committed to ensuring that those I connect with or support have the similar opportunities so they can find their home.

A few years ago I gave my sons a book to complete as their Mother's Day gift to me: *A Whole Book About Things I Love About Mom* by Em & Friends. It was a beautiful, eye-opening exercise, as I truly saw their version of me through their words. Through the eyes of my fourteen-year-old son, I am still a superhero; my ten-year-old son has realized that I am not just his mom but a person; and my passion for working and helping others in the workplace inspires my seven-year-old son. Plus, dancing is big in our house! I am fairly confident that if you were to ask my past and current colleagues the same questions, superheroes and dancing would also probably come up in discussion.

So, I leave you with this: no matter where your story takes you to balance the limited hours in a day, either to build the business of your dreams as an entrepreneur to dedicate available time to your family and as a mother, or to find a home in an organization that provides you with the opportunity to use your strengths and passions to make an impact within the structure, bring your whole self, your authentic self, to whatever you do. Eventually, the light will shine, and you'll find your way. And perhaps one day you'll be the shining light for someone else as they navigate their own journey to find their way home.

Works CITED

Introduction by Sabrina Greer

Field of Dreams directed by Phil Alden Robinson. Gordon, 1989.

Chapter 1 by Sabrina Greer

Pauline Boss PhD. *Ambiguous Loss: Learning to Live with Unresolved Grief.* Harvard University Press, 1999.

Chapter 9 by Apryl Jennings

David A. Cooper. *The Mystical Kabbalah: Judaism's Ancient System for Mystical Enlightenment through Meditation and Contemplation.* Sounds True, 2001.

Chapter 12 by Lindsay Grace

Rhonda Bryne. *The Secret.* Atria Books, 2006.

The Secret directed by Drew Heriot. Prime Time Productions, 2006.

Chapter 14 by Jenny Bitner

A Course in Miracles. https://acim.org/acim/en, accessed July 6, 2023.

Chapter 15 by Nicole Campagna

Em and Friends. *A Whole Book About Things I Love About Mom.* Knock Knock Books, 2019.

SOUL SEED
L E G A C Y · H O U S E

At Soul Seed Legacy House, we help thought leaders
and creative entrepreneurs capture their vision in the
form of nonfiction books, journals, workbooks,
affirmation cards, and personal growth products.

Our mission is to help our authors grow and scale a
platform far beyond the book, protect their soul's work,
and turn their message into a legacy!

www.sslegacyhouse.com

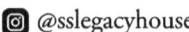 @sslegacyhouse

www.ingramcontent.com/pod-product-compliance
Lightning Source LLC
Chambersburg PA
CBHW051618120626

46551CB00014B/1844

9 781998 754335